Fast Facts

Fast Facts: Breast Cancer

Fourth edition

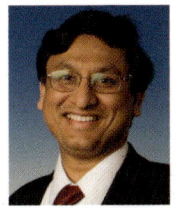

Jayant S Vaidya MBBS MS DNB FRCS PhD FRCS(Gen)
Senior Lecturer and Consultant Surgeon
Research Department of Surgery
Division of Surgery and Interventional Science
University College London, UK
(www.jayantvaidya.org)

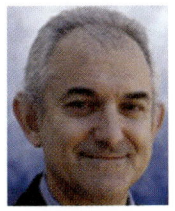

David Joseph MBBS FRACR MRACMA
Clinical Professor
Medical Director, Cancer Division
and Director of Radiation Oncology
Sir Charles Gairdner Hospital
Perth, Australia

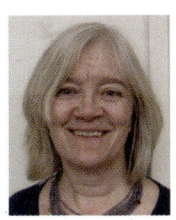

Alison Jones MD FRCP
Consultant Medical Oncologist
Royal Free Hospital, London, UK

Declaration of Independence
This book is as balanced and as practical as we can make it.
Ideas for improvement are always welcome: feedback@fastfacts.com

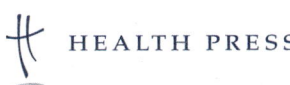

Fast Facts – Breast Cancer
First published 1998; second edition 2002; third edition 2005
Fourth edition June 2010

Text © 2010 Jayant S Vaidya, David Joseph and Alison Jones
© 2010 in this edition Health Press Limited
Health Press Limited, Elizabeth House, Queen Street, Abingdon,
Oxford OX14 3LN, UK
Tel: +44 (0)1235 523233
Fax: +44 (0)1235 523238

Book orders can be placed by telephone or via the website.
For regional distributors or to order via the website, please go to: www.fastfacts.com
For telephone orders, please call +44 (0)1752 202301 (UK and Europe),
1 800 247 6553 (USA, toll free), +1 419 281 1802 (Americas) or
+61 (0)2 9698 7755 (Asia–Pacific).

Fast Facts is a trademark of Health Press Limited.

All rights reserved. No part of this publication may be reproduced, stored in a
retrieval system, or transmitted in any form or by any means, electronic, mechanical,
photocopying, recording or otherwise, without the express permission of the
publisher.

The rights of Jayant S Vaidya, David Joseph and Alison Jones to be identified as the
authors of this work have been asserted in accordance with the Copyright, Designs &
Patents Act 1988 Sections 77 and 78.

The publisher and the authors have made every effort to ensure the accuracy of this
book, but cannot accept responsibility for any errors or omissions.

For all drugs, please consult the product labeling approved in your country for
prescribing information.

Registered names, trademarks, etc. used in this book, even when not marked as such,
are not to be considered unprotected by law.

A CIP catalogue record for this title is available from the British Library.

ISBN 978-1-905832-78-1

Vaidya JS (Jayant)
Fast Facts – Breast Cancer/
Jayant S Vaidya, David Joseph, Alison Jones

Medical illustrations by Dee McLean, London, UK
Typesetting and page layout by Zed, Oxford, UK
Printed by Latimer Trend & Company Limited, Plymouth, UK

Text printed with vegetable inks on biodegradable and
recyclable paper manufactured using elemental chlorine
free (ECF) wood pulp from well-managed forests.

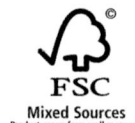

Introduction	5
Risk factors	7
Perception of risk	19
Pathophysiology	28
Diagnosis	47
Local control of primary tumor	65
Adjuvant therapy	83
Follow-up and rehabilitation	106
Management of advanced cancer	111
Clinical trials	126
Future trends	131
Useful addresses	136
Index	138

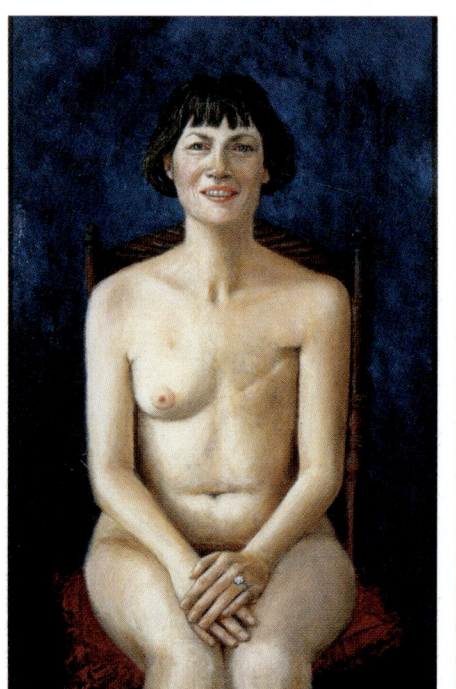 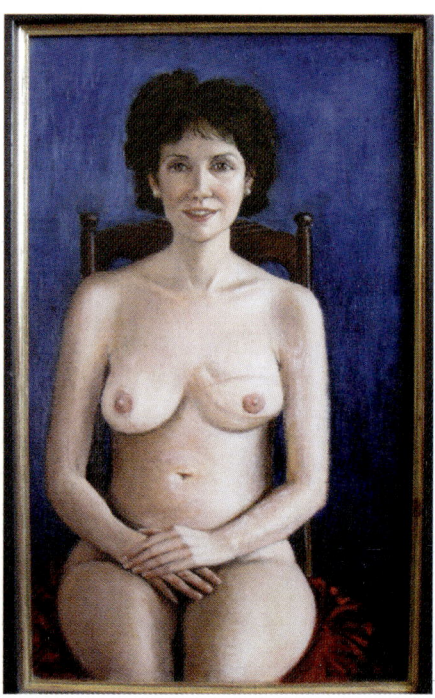

'There is life after mastectomy' and 'Reconstruction'. Portraits by Heath Rosselli, reproduced by kind permission of the artist.

Introduction

We are currently in the most exciting period for the management of breast cancer. Great progress has been made and is accruing at an ever-increasing rate.

In most parts of the world, mortality from breast cancer has been reduced dramatically over the last 10 years. A large proportion of this improvement can be attributed to the changing paradigms about the disease and new treatments, proven in randomized clinical trials and consequently applied widely. More precise diagnosis, refined treatments and advances in adjuvant systemic treatment are being adopted in the general population.

The past few years have offered the beginnings of a fundamental change. Our conceptual understanding of malignancy is evolving from that of a pathological entity to that of a regulatory process. As a consequence, the period for intervention extends from the time preventative measures are taken, years before a clinical tumor is likely to appear, to long after local resection of an obvious mass. This has significant implications for both the patient and the healthcare system, as the net effect is to increase the number of patients and extend the period of follow-up.

There has been an explosion in information technology and easier access to information for patients and their families and medical advisors. Patients can now be more knowledgeable and assume a more active role in their medical management.

Multidisciplinary management of breast cancer is now the standard of care. The evidence for this is mainly circumstantial; however, there is some evidence that a certain minimum volume is required to maintain a high quality of outcome.

Cancer centers are no longer just venues for treatment, but are becoming regional resources offering guidance in decision-making, leading innovations in treatment, education and training, as well as collecting valuable data for evaluation. The need to balance choices is a theme repeated throughout the book, and *Fast Facts: Breast Cancer* attempts to provide a context for putting the risks and benefits into perspective. The purpose of this book is to sort out the facts from the fancies and fallacies, and to provide the busy clinician or clinical nurse specialist with rapid access to information that will make their difficult and delicate task that much easier. We owe it to our patients to provide them with comprehensive care and must make every effort to maintain their integration within the community throughout the course of a chronic illness.

1 Risk factors

Breast cancer is the most common form of cancer among women in industrialized countries, accounting for about 18% of all female cancers. Although mortality is declining in some areas, breast cancer remains the leading cause of death among women aged 35–55 years. In the UK, for example, it causes about 13 000 deaths each year, and about 35 000 new cases are diagnosed annually, while in the USA, there are about 217 500 new cases and 40 580 deaths.

It is important to recognize that the oft-repeated statistic that 1 in 10 women get breast cancer can be misinterpreted, especially by young women. The absolute risk of being diagnosed with breast cancer is about 1.5% at 40–50 years of age, 2.5% at 50–60 years of age and reaches 1 in 12 only when all those up to 100 years of age are included.

Classic epidemiological studies repeated worldwide have established risk associations with breast cancer. These associations have been bolstered by tissue and animal studies. The following observations, which were made before the advent of contemporary molecular genetics, continue to hold true.

The incidence of breast cancer increases with age; approximately 50% of breast cancers occur in women aged 50–64 years, and a further 30% occur in women over the age of 70 years. The incidence also shows marked geographical variations; in general, the highest incidences are seen in Western countries, and the lowest in Asian and African countries (Figure 1.1). This illustrates the importance of environmental risk factors, as women from low-risk countries, such as Japan, who emigrate to higher-risk countries ultimately develop the higher risk associated with their new country. Genetic factors are also important, however, as the natural history of breast cancer appears to vary between populations. In Japanese women, for example, the disease appears to develop earlier and to take a more benign course than in Western women, whereas black African women also develop breast cancer earlier, but suffer from much more aggressive disease. Also of striking significance is the rapid rise in incidence in some European countries,

Fast Facts: Breast Cancer

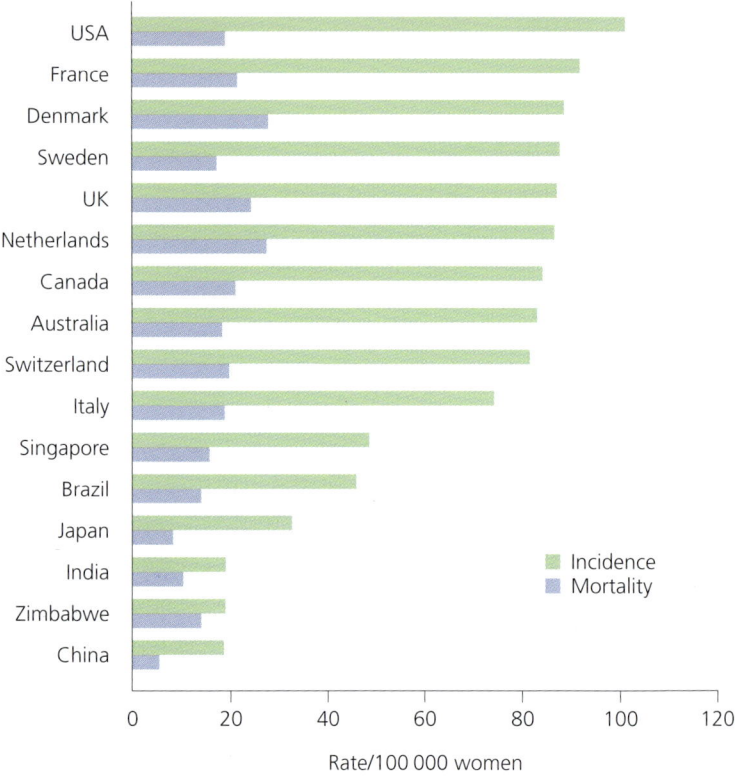

Figure 1.1 Breast cancer incidence and mortality show marked geographical variations. Data from Ferlay J, Bray F, Pisani P, Parkin DM. *GLOBOCAN 2002. Cancer Incidence, Mortality and Prevalence Worldwide.* International Agency for Research on Cancer CancerBase No. 5, version 2.0. Lyon: IARC Press, 2004.

such as Spain, as their prosperity begins to approach that of the European Union as a whole. In addition to age and geographical origin, numerous risk-modifying associations have been identified (Table 1.1).

Age

Age is by far the greatest risk factor for breast cancer in women. Of the approximately 60% of breast cancers for which identifiable risk factors can be found, age accounts for more than half.

TABLE 1.1
Factors influencing the risk of breast cancer

	High risk	Low risk
	Relative risk 1.1–2.0	
Age at first full-term pregnancy	≥ 30 years	< 20 years
Age at menarche	< 12 years	> 14 years
Age at menopause	≥ 55 years	< 45 years
Obesity (postmenopausal)	Obese (BMI > 30)	Thin (BMI = 20–25)
Alcohol/day	Relative risk: ≤ 1 drink = 1.08; 1–2 drinks = 1.21; and > 2 drinks = 1.38	No alcohol
Level of physical activity	Low	Moderate or greater
Parity (postmenopausal)	Nulliparous	Multiparous
Breast-feeding (premenopausal)	None	Several years
Hormonal contraceptives	Yes	No
Hormone replacement therapy	Yes	No
Socioeconomic status	High	Low
Place of residence	Urban	Rural
Race/ethnicity		
Breast cancer at age < 40 years	White	Asian
Breast cancer at age ≥ 40 years	Black	Asian
Religion	Jewish	Mormon, Seventh-day Adventist

CONTINUED

TABLE 1.1 (CONTINUED)

	High risk	Low risk
Relative risk 2.1–4.0		
Nodular densities on mammogram (postmenopausal)	> 75% of breast volume	Parenchyma composed entirely of fat
One first-degree relative with breast cancer	Yes	No
Biopsy-confirmed atypical hyperplasia	Yes	No
High-dose radiation to chest	Yes	No
Ovariectomy before age 35 years	No	Yes
Relative risk > 4.0		
Age	> 50 years	< 30 years
Place of birth	North America, Northern Europe	Asia, Africa
Two first-degree relatives with breast cancer diagnosed at an early age	Yes	No
History of cancer in one breast	Yes	No

BMI, body mass index

Family history

The risk of breast cancer is increased two- to three-fold in women with a first-degree relative with breast cancer; the risk is also increased, but to a lesser extent, in women with a second-degree relative who is affected. The risk is particularly high if:
- the affected relative is on the maternal side of the family
- two first-degree relatives are affected
- the relative has bilateral breast cancer
- the relative's cancer was diagnosed before the age of 50 years.

Overall, 10–15% of breast cancers are attributable to family history, and half of these can be attributed to specific susceptibility genes. The genetics of breast cancer are discussed more fully on pages 15–17.

Demography

The risk of breast cancer is increased in women from higher socioeconomic classes, and in women living in urban areas. However, women from higher socioeconomic classes almost uniformly have a better prognosis, even when matched for disease stage and treatment. This may well be due to inherent molecular differences (e.g. p53), but the direction of causality is arguable.

Menses

The risk of breast cancer is increased in women who begin to menstruate at an early age (< 12 years) or who undergo the menopause at a relatively advanced age (> 55 years). Conversely, the risk is reduced in women in whom menarche is delayed, or who undergo bilateral ovariectomy before the age of about 35 years. This may partly explain the protective effect of early first pregnancy, as it has been suggested that it is the number of menstrual cycles before the first pregnancy that ultimately determines the risk of breast cancer. Perhaps an early first pregnancy allows an early complete maturation of the ductoglandular tissue, rather than leaving it in a less differentiated state that is perhaps more susceptible to environmental carcinogenic factors. Thus, in Western countries with the highest incidences of breast cancer, menstruation typically begins at about the age of 12 years, but the average age at first pregnancy is about 25 years. By contrast, in less developed countries, menstruation may not begin until the age of 17–18 years and the first pregnancy may have occurred by the age of 20 years, thus exposing the breasts to fewer cycles of aborted attempts at full differentiation.

Pregnancy

Age at first full-term pregnancy appears to be the most important factor influencing hormonal status and thereby reducing the risk of breast cancer. For women who have their first child before the age of about 25 years, the risk of breast cancer is approximately half that of women who have their first child after 30 years of age; a woman in the latter category has the same risk as someone who remains childless. Furthermore, multiparous postmenopausal women have a lower risk of breast cancer than nulliparous women. There is some suggestion that pregnancy-associated hypertension is associated with reduced risk and diethylstilbestrol exposure of the mother with increased risk.

It was suggested that interruption of the process of maturation of ductoglandular tissue, either early (spontaneous or induced abortion) or late (premature birth), leaves a population of unstable cells, thus increasing the risk of cancer. However, a large meta-analysis of 53 studies and 83 000 women in 16 countries found no increased risk of breast cancer in women who had had an abortion, largely refuting this hypothesis.

It is interesting that full-term pregnancy is associated with lower mammographic breast density; mammographic breast density has recently been established as an independent predictor of breast cancer risk, though a complete explanation for this finding is still being sought.

Breast-feeding

The effect of breast-feeding has been difficult to establish, mainly because the duration of lactation in early studies was short. Only prolonged lactation has been found to independently reduce the risk of breast cancer (by about 4% per year of breast-feeding).

Diet and obesity

Obesity is associated with an increased risk of breast cancer in postmenopausal women. This increased risk may be due to conversion of adrenal androgens to estrogens in adipose tissue.

High consumption of animal fats has also been linked to breast cancer. However, a meta-analysis of cohort studies involving over 330 000 women found no evidence for an association between the relative risk of breast cancer and dietary fat intake. Nevertheless, a randomized trial in early-stage breast cancer has shown that a reduction in dietary fat intake reduced the risk of breast cancer recurrence.

Folate supplements may reduce the risk of breast cancer; however, the Women's Health Initiative observational study found that, contrary to the findings of previous studies, folate did not attenuate the increased risk from alcohol consumption.

Recent evidence from a study of the Chinese diet suggests that it is the high intake of phytoestrogens in vegetables and grains (soy isoflavones) rather than low fat intake that exerts a protective effect. A clinical trial examining the effect of food additives derived from the oriental diet on the prevention of breast cancer has therefore been proposed.

A diet based predominantly on bread and pasta is associated with an increased risk of breast cancer compared with a diet based predominantly on fruit and vegetables.

Oral contraceptives

A recent meta-analysis involving over 150 000 women has examined the influence of oral contraceptive (OC) use on the risk of breast cancer. The relative risk was slightly increased (1.24) in women who had used OCs within 10 years, but no excess risk was seen in those who had used OCs more than 10 years previously. The risk is particularly high when OCs are taken before the first full-term pregnancy. Although the incidence of breast cancer was increased in OC users, mortality from the disease remained constant because the cancers tended to be of a more favorable type.

The slight increase in risk associated with OCs should, however, be viewed in the context of women's health in general. It is very likely that OCs substantially diminish the risk of ovarian and endometrial carcinoma. They are also highly effective as a form of contraception and as a means of relieving menses-related morbidity. There is no evidence that current formulations of OCs affect breast cancer risk. However, this will not be known for certain for another 30 years, since the cohort of women who have taken the pill (particularly low-dose preparations) are only now reaching the age at which they are at risk of breast cancer.

Hormone replacement therapy

Several large observational studies have clearly shown that hormone replacement therapy (HRT) increases the risk of developing breast cancer. Women taking HRT also have greater breast density on mammography, making it more difficult to detect small cancers. A recent sudden fall in the incidence of breast cancer in the USA has been attributed to the reduction in HRT use by women after the results of these larges studies were published. However, this fall has been rather too soon to reflect changes in HRT use and is not seen in all countries, most notably in Scotland where about 80% of the population undergo mammographic screening. It has been suggested (by the author) that HRT probably promotes the growth of only symptomatic cancers.

It is currently considered that HRT is only acceptable to control significant menopausal symptoms (such as hot flashes) following full discussion about the risks. It is important to remember that HRT probably does *not* confer any cardiovascular benefit and better drugs are available for preventing or treating osteoporosis.

Alcohol consumption

The consumption of approximately 15 g or more of alcohol (equivalent to 2–3 glasses of wine or measures of spirits) each day increases the risk of breast cancer by about 50%. This may be attributable to reduced hepatic estrogen metabolism. For every additional drink (or 5 g of alcohol) consumed per day, it is estimated that 11 additional breast cancers will occur per 1000 women. The relative risks (compared with lifelong abstainers) are 1.08 (95% confidence interval [CI] 0.95–1.22) for those who have less than 1 drink per day, 1.21 (95% CI 1.05–1.40; $p = 0.01$) for those who have 1–2 drinks per day and 1.38 (95% CI 1.13–1.68; $p = 0.002$) for those who have 3 or more drinks per day. There is clear evidence that regular drinking also increases the risk of recurrence, as well as contralateral breast cancer, in breast cancer survivors.

Exercise

Research, including several large studies, has provided good evidence that exercise and physical activity reduce the risk of both premenopausal and postmenopausal breast cancer, as well as the risk of recurrence after a diagnosis of breast cancer. Weight reduction is also associated with a reduced risk. Regular exercise could be considered as one of the easiest (at least in theory), most modifiable risk factors for breast cancer and, indeed, has a large beneficial effect in absolute terms, apart from its cardiac and metabolic benefits.

Mammographic breast density

There is increasing and compelling evidence that mammographic breast density correlates directly with the risk of breast cancer, with a relative risk of up to 4 between the most dense and least dense breasts. While this finding is not very well explained, it remains an independent risk factor. The addition of breast density significantly improves the discriminatory power of conventional risk-predicting models. Interestingly, a recent study found that recent alcohol intake, particularly of beer and white wine (as opposed to red wine), correlated directly with mammographic breast density; another study found that women living in urban areas have a higher breast density.

Genetics

With the rise of modern genetics research, a subcellular and molecular understanding of familial factors in breast cancer is emerging. New technologies have allowed detailed comparisons to be made between the chromosome patterns of 'normal' populations and those at high risk, which meant, initially, women with very strong family histories. From these studies, the first genes that were strongly associated with breast cancer were identified, notably the breast cancer susceptibility genes, *BRCA1* (17q21) and *BRCA2* (13q14). More recent research in Ashkenazi Jewish populations, which have a high prevalence of mutations in these genes, suggests that *BRCA1* and *BRCA2* are associated with a high risk of breast cancer, even in the absence of a family history. Mutations in these genes are implicated in approximately 4% of all breast cancers and in up to 25% of patients diagnosed before the age of 40 years; they are also linked to ovarian cancers. The breast cancer risk associated with mutations in *BRCA2* appears less than that with mutations in *BRCA1*, but the presence of the gene mutation carries additional, smaller risks of male breast and prostate cancers, and perhaps others.

Neither *BRCA1* nor *BRCA2* should be considered 'breast-cancer specific' in the sense that a single mutation leads directly to disease, as in sickle-cell disease, for example. Both genes represent large segments on specific chromosomes where a number of deviations from the base sequence of DNA in the normal population are concentrated. It is believed that some of these changes result in inappropriate cellular proliferation, or are linked to a failure of DNA repair as a final common pathway. *BRCA1* does not appear to be a classic tumor suppressor gene and, somewhat paradoxically, it is not associated with sporadic cancers. However, there is some evidence that the gene may act in a novel way to suppress the function of other inhibitors of proliferation.

The BRCA proteins appear to play a subtle role in the central control of the sex-steroid-regulated pathways, which is in keeping with the emerging understanding of cancer as a dynamic regulatory control disease. Normal BRCA1 appears to suppress the signaling of mammary epithelial cells by the estrogen receptor. BRCA2 is functionally related, but distinct. Whether the genetic mutations predestine the cancer or merely facilitate malignant transformation is unknown. Recent data from twin studies suggest that the mutated genes exert their influence very early, and set the context for the development of breast cancer in response to a hormonal stimulus that might otherwise be benign. Moreover, changes in *BRCA2* do not appear to be restricted to breast cancer. One of the genes closely associated with Fanconi's anemia appears to be identical to *BRCA2*. A fascinating postulate supported by early data is that the *BRCA2* mutation inherited from one parent leads to an elevated risk of breast and prostate cancer, but when inherited from both parents leads to a pediatric blood disorder.

BRCA1 and *BRCA2* are not the only genes implicated in breast cancer. One of the common DNA-sequence variants that confer a small increase in breast cancer risk is *CHEK2*. It is a component of the machinery that recognizes and repairs damaged DNA, and seems to activate *BRCA1*. Germline mutations in *TP53*, which encodes tumor protein p53 (Li–Fraumeni syndrome), usually lead to childhood cancers, but girls who reach adulthood have a risk of breast cancer as high as 90%. *EMSY*, a newly identified gene that is overexpressed in sporadic breast cancers, produces a protein that interacts with BRCA2.

Although our understanding is rudimentary, a general concept emerges. Genes represent predisposition. The internal hormonal and regulatory milieu of the body, and life events such as diet, drugs, pregnancies and levels of activity are stimuli in a dynamic homeostatic process. The interaction between predisposition and provocation is

when malignancy appears. It is reasonable to hypothesize that genetic mutations have an influence beyond susceptibility. Even in these early days, there is evidence that gene expression signatures can predict:
- risk of disease
- relapse and survival risk
- patterns of recurrence
- response to therapy.

When these regulatory pathways are better understood, establishing the point at which intervention is necessary will pose a substantial challenge and will profoundly influence our preventive and treatment strategies in the future.

Methylation profiles

In addition to genes, there is increasing evidence that epigenetic mechanisms (chemical reactions that switch part of the genome on or off at specific times or locations) can significantly influence breast cancer risk. A correlation between certain methylation profiles and conventional risk factors for breast cancer has been shown. Research is ongoing into how epigenetic profiling may enable the identification of women at higher risk within conventional risk stratifications. It is also examining whether any intervention that changes such methylation profiles alters the risk of developing breast cancer.

Key points – risk factors

- Age is the greatest risk factor.
- Mutations in the breast cancer genes *BRCA1* and *BRCA2* denote high risk, but account for only a small proportion of cancers. Mutations in several other genes, including *CHEK2*, *TP53* and *EMSY*, are involved.
- Hormonal factors, such as menstrual and obstetric history, and exogenous hormones affect the risk of breast cancer.
- Diet, exercise, alcohol and smoking are modifiable risk factors.
- Mammographic breast density is an independent and powerful risk factor that remains to be fully explained.

Key references

Collaborative Group on Hormonal Factors in Breast Cancer. Breast cancer and abortion: collaborative reanalysis of data from 53 epidemiological studies, including 83 000 women with breast cancer from 16 countries. *Lancet* 2004; 363:1007–16.

Cummings SR, Tice JA, Bauer S et al. Prevention of breast cancer in postmenopausal women: approaches to estimating and reducing risk. *J Natl Cancer Inst* 2009;101:384–98.

Flom JD, Ferris JS, Tehranifar P, Terry MB. Alcohol intake over the life course and mammographic density. *Breast Cancer Res Treat* 2009;117:643–51.

Hughes-Davis L, Huntsman D, Ruas M et al. *EMSY* links the *BRCA2* pathway to sporadic breast and ovarian cancer. *Cell* 2003;115: 523–35.

Levi F, Luchini F, Negri E, La Vecchia C. The fall in breast cancer mortality in Europe. *Eur J Cancer* 2001;37:1409–12.

Minelli C, Abrams KR, Sutton AJ et al. Benefits and harms associated with hormone replacement therapy: clinical decision analysis. *BMJ* 2004;328:371–5.

Neiburgs H. Molecular genetics and cancer: the role of *BRCA1* and *BRCA2*. *Womens Oncol Rev* 2002;2:19–29.

Saunders CM, Baum M. Breast cancer and pregnancy: a review. *J R Soc Med* 1993;86:162–5.

Thompson WD. Genetic epidemiology of breast cancer. *Cancer* 1994;74(suppl):279–87.

Van de Vijver MJ, He YD, van't Veer LJ et al. A gene-expression signature as a predictor of survival in breast cancer. *N Engl J Med* 2002;347:1999–2009.

Wooster R, Weber BL. Breast and ovarian cancer. *N Engl J Med* 2003; 348:2339–47.

2 Perception of risk

Despite the current preoccupation with the notion of risk, it is a poorly understood concept, and one that is more questionably acted on in public policy and healthcare. Breast cancer in all its aspects is under intense scrutiny, and three areas in particular are controversial: screening, adjuvant therapy, and the treatment of advanced disease. Moreover, the clinical trials process, which is essential to increasing our understanding of cancer, is all about risk.

Three definitions form the basis of risk assessment:
- risk or odds
- consequence or harm
- balance or comparison.

Risk is a measurement of likelihood, or how often an event takes place. It is a proportional quantity. Implicit in the concept is a comparison of the number of times an event might occur with the number of times it actually does occur. For example, if the risk of falling off a mountain is estimated to be 1/10 000, then for every 10 000 individual mountain-climbing excursions, one person falls. The term 'risk' carries a negative connotation, though in fact it is intended to be a neutral term; conversely 'odds' has a more positive implication (e.g. the odds of winning).

Explaining the concept of risk

People have some sense of the total effect of a specific risk. However, there is no metric for identifying, summing and weighing all hazards and consequences. The event risks are constantly changing. The consequences vary with time and circumstance, and individuals making personal choices change their internal evaluation strategies over time. The best approach is to give a clear explanation of the basic principles and to set individual risk/consequence discussions in the context of the other hazards that exist. There is no single risk that exists in isolation.

Thus, when explaining the concept of risk to a patient, there are a number of points worth considering.

- It is helpful to set risk in context, by comparing the risk of breast cancer with that of trauma or heart disease: for example, for non-smoking women, the 10-year risks of death from breast cancer and heart disease are similar until the age of 60 (typically ≤ 1%). Past age 60, heart disease becomes the single largest cause of death. From age 40 onwards, current women smokers are much more likely to die from heart disease or lung cancer than from breast cancer (the risk for death from heart disease or lung cancer being at least five times that from breast cancer after the age of 55). The overall risk of dying from breast cancer lies between 1% and 2% from 40 to 50 years of age and between 2% and 3% from 50 to 60 years.
- The distinction between risk and consequence should be clarified (see below).
- Risk is a proportional quantity. A doubling of a very small risk may be far less worrisome than a 5% increase in a very large risk.
- All interventions, including doing nothing, involve a trade-off of risks.

Consequence or harm represents the severity of the effect of the risk event should it happen, which also carries a negative connotation. The total effect of a given risk is the product of the risk and the consequence. Numerous studies have shown that people tend to pay more attention to negative consequences than positive ones, particularly when the former are seen as gruesome, refractory to treatment and poorly understood.

There is an important corollary to the notion that no risk exists in isolation. Conceptually, the proper approach to the assessment of risk would be to sum the product of all possible risks and their consequences. In reality, this is very difficult to do and, as a result, there is often an exaggerated focus on rare, potentially dramatic, adverse consequences.

Balance or comparison is another vital principle. The concept of relative or proportionate risk underlies all of medicine. When considering individual hazards, it is important to make the distinction between the proportionate risk (i.e. the ratio of events taking place with or without intervention) and the absolute risk (i.e. the likelihood of the event as a proportion of the entire population at risk). A small proportionate advance against a high-frequency risk may be of greater consequence than a large advance against a rare risk. This issue becomes significant in discussions about adjuvant therapy for breast cancer.

Screening

Breast cancer screening, for an individual woman, is an exercise in understanding the basic principle of risk – the likelihood of an adverse event. Women generally grossly overestimate their risk of developing breast cancer and, as a consequence, overrate the benefits that may be gained from screening.

A 2009 Cochrane review found that for every 2000 women invited for screening for 10 years, there is one fewer death (10 vs 11 deaths), while 10 additional cancers (44 vs 34) are diagnosed – cancers which would have otherwise not become clinically evident in the woman's lifetime.

Describing the risk of developing breast cancer as 1 in 10–12 is true, yet unhelpful, because this figure is the cumulative lifetime risk. In real terms, the background risk for women between the ages of 30 and 50 years is about 1 per 1000 per year or 2% on aggregate whereas, before the age of 30 years, breast cancer is exceptionally rare. Between 50 and 70 years of age, which is the period when mammographic screening is most often recommended, the risk goes up to about 2 per 1000 per year, which is approximately 2% on aggregate in the first decade of the menopause, rising steeply thereafter, with about one-third of all reported breast cancers occurring in the 70–85-year age group.

It is important to explain what any increase in relative risk means in real terms. For example, if a woman finds out that she has a relative risk of breast cancer that is twice that of the normal population, she may understandably panic and assume that she has a one in six chance of dying of the disease within the foreseeable future. Yet if she is 30 years old her risk doubles to 2/1000/year or 2% in a decade, which might seem insignificant against the other risks of living in a modern urban society. Furthermore, any increases in the relative risks are not distributed symmetrically throughout a woman's lifetime, but tend to occur before the age of 60, after which the risk levels return to normal. Women counseled in this way are often comforted and do not feel the need for unnecessary mammographic screening, and are unlikely to contemplate prophylactic mastectomy, which is a growth industry in the USA.

Genetic testing. The identification of some mutations in the breast cancer genes (*BRCA1*, *BRCA2*) among women with a poor family history is, of course, a different matter altogether. Early data suggested that the breast cancer risk of women who carried the mutation could be as high as 85%, but more recent data from Europe seem to indicate that the risk is of the order of 50%. The potential advantage of genetic testing in women with very strong family histories is that a negative result would effectively reduce the woman's risk to the level in the background population, and thus alleviate much concern and perhaps unnecessary intervention. On the other hand, a positive result might lead to more rational decisions about prophylactic mastectomy. Individual risk can be estimated from models built from epidemiological data, such as the Claus or Gale models.

Treatment of early breast cancer

Proportional risk is perhaps the most important concept to arise from the many trials of systemic (adjuvant) therapy for early breast cancer. Each type of treatment reduces the risk of breast cancer recurrence by a relatively constant proportion. Thus, in premenopausal women, chemotherapy reduces the risk of recurrence by 33% and ovariectomy by about 25%, while in postmenopausal women, tamoxifen reduces the risk by about 40%. Thus, the benefit for a given woman in absolute terms depends on both the effect of treatment on the relative risk and the underlying individual risk factors. Fundamental to interpreting estimates of benefit is the understanding that the proportion being calculated relates to the number of adverse events, not the number of individuals at risk. For example, a premenopausal woman with a 1.5-cm tumor without nodal involvement may have a 10-year risk of recurrence of 10%. If adjuvant chemotherapy produces a relative risk reduction of about 30% then, in absolute terms, the patient gains 30% of the 10% chance of living disease-free for 10 years, which is about 3%. On the other hand, if the same woman has four nodes involved, her 10-year risk of recurrence is about 50%. The treatment offers a 30% relative risk reduction, leading to an absolute benefit of 30% of 50%: a 15% decrease in the probability of recurrence within 10 years.

There are two important further considerations. First, the data from which these recommendations derive are generally specific for the risk of breast cancer; competing adverse risks, including the toxicity of treatment, are not considered. In that respect, the data may overestimate benefit. Secondly, in contrast to the benefit being calculated against the number of adverse events, the toxicity of treatment affects the entire population treated and not solely those who experience an adverse event. Thus, if the risk of an adverse event is 25%, then 1 in 4 of those who receive the treatment will experience the effect. If only 3 in 100 benefit from a reduction in the recurrence risk, it might be said that 25 people experience side effects in order that 3 accrue a benefit. Clearly, the greater the recurrence risk, the more likely people will be willing to accept toxicity. These are complex issues that cannot be discussed fully in this limited overview. Figure 2.1 provides some clarification of the central concepts relating to the risks and benefits of treatment, and computer software is now available to help women make informed choices in selecting adjuvant systemic therapy based on this principle.

Advanced disease

At present, treatment of recurrent or advanced disease is not likely to extend survival in most patients. The risk discussion thus becomes one of comparing and contrasting consequences. In this setting, the baseline consequences are symptoms or closely anticipated symptoms, and the consequence of intervention is side effects. The risk-management strategy becomes one of direct trade-off, namely 'paying' for a diminution of disease-related morbidity with treatment-related morbidity. In some respects the calculation is more difficult, since the 'event' being sought is not discrete (as in a recurrence), but an alteration in symptoms or signs.

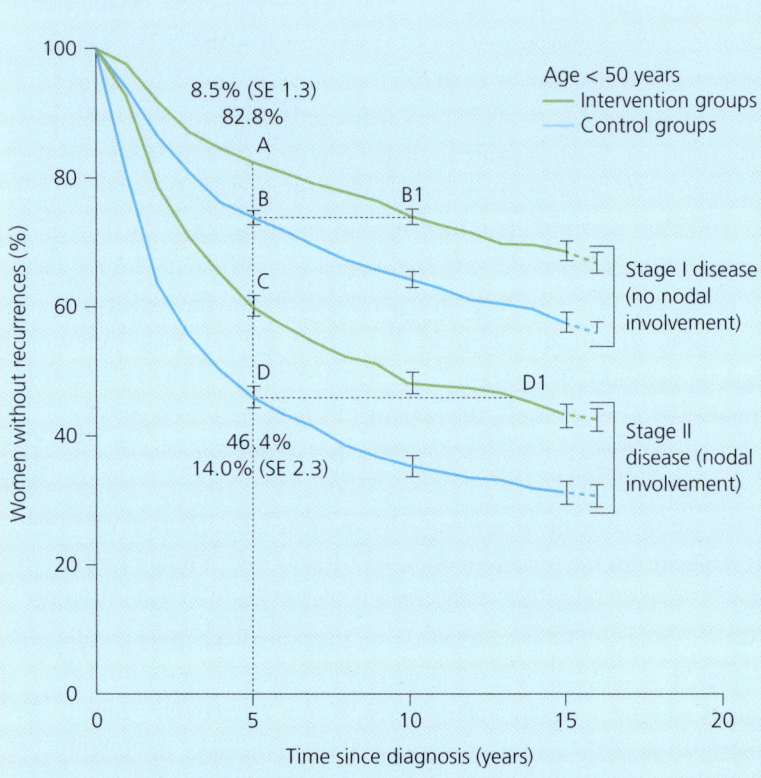

Figure 2.1 This figure is intended to clarify concepts relating to the risks and benefits of treatment for early stage breast cancer. The figure is derived from the Early Breast Cancer Trialists' Collaborative Group Overview, and is intended as an example.

The two upper curves represent women without nodal involvement (stage I). The lower pair represents those with evidence of nodal involvement. In both pairs, the upper curve is the intervention arm, the lower the control arm. The plots are arithmetic, though these data are often presented in semilogarithmic form.

For this example, consider the results at 5 years. The issue is the number of 'events', meaning recurrences, which have been prevented or delayed at this point. For women with stage I disease, point **B** is the

proportion of women whose tumors recurred without treatment, 25.8% (100 − 74.2). Point **A** is the proportion who had recurrences despite treatment, 17.2% (100 − 82.8). The risk reduction can be presented two ways:
- as a proportion of those whose tumors recurred without treatment, calculated as (25.8 − 17.2)/25.8 = 0.3333 or 33.3%
- as a proportion of the treatment population, sometimes called the absolute benefit, calculated as the risk without treatment minus the risk with treatment, in this case 82.8 − 74.2 = 8.6%.

For stage II women, the calculations are as follows. Point **C** represents recurrence in women receiving treatment, 39.6% (100 − 60.4), and point **D** the recurrence rate in the control arm, 53.6% (100 − 46.4). Again, the risk reduction can be presented two ways:
- as a proportion of those whose tumors recurred without treatment, calculated as (53.6 − 39.6)/53.6 = 0.261 or 26.1%
- as the absolute benefit, in this case 53.6 − 39.6 = 14%.

The crucial message is the distinction between proportionate and absolute benefit. In this case, the proportionate benefit for intervention in stage I disease appears greater than that in stage II (33.3% vs 26.1%). However, in absolute terms, stage II patients derive a greater benefit (14% vs 8.6%). The explanation is that there are more recurrences to start with in stage II disease.

Finally, the horizontal distances B to B1 and D to D1 are occasionally used to estimate the 'time gained' by virtue of the treatment. This is a controversial analysis, in part because it assumes that those patients who have recurrences are otherwise biologically identical to those who do not, and that the difference is solely due to treatment. Given that there are significant numbers of women whose cancers would not have recurred, even without intervention, that assumption may not be entirely true.

Key points – perception of risk

- Risk is a poorly understood concept – nothing is risk free.
- Risk measures the likelihood that an event will take place.
- Risk is a proportional quantity; change in risk can be expressed in absolute or relative terms.
- Consequence represents the severity of effect of an event.
- Decision making involves balancing of risks.
- Correct decisions about lifestyle choices, screening and selection of adjuvant systemic therapy depend on the understanding of these issues and making value judgments.

Key references

Becher H, Chang-Claude J. Estimating disease risks for individuals with a given family history in different populations with an application to breast cancer. *Genet Epidemiol* 1996;13:229–42.

Benichou J, Gale MH, Mulvihill JJ. Graphs to estimate an individualized risk of breast cancer. *J Clin Oncol* 1996;14:103–10.

Bianchi S, Palli D, Galli M, Zampi G. Benign breast disease and cancer risk. *Crit Rev Oncol Hematol* 1993;15:221–42.

Black WC, Nease RF, Tosteson AVA. Perceptions of breast cancer risk and screening effectiveness in women younger than 50 years of age. *J Natl Cancer Inst* 1995;87:720–3.

Claus EB, Risch N, Thompson WD. Autosomal dominant inheritance of early-onset breast cancer. Implications for risk prediction. *Cancer* 1994;73:643–51.

Colditz GA, Hankinson SE, Hunter DJ et al. The use of estrogens and progestins and the risk of breast cancer in post-menopausal women. *N Engl J Med* 1995;332:1589–93.

Cuzick J, Powles T, Veronesi U et al. Overview of the main outcomes in breast-cancer prevention trials. *Lancet* 2003;361:296–300.

Dupont WD, Page DL. Risk factors for breast cancer in women with proliferative disease. *N Engl J Med* 1985;312:146–51.

Fisher B, Costantino JP, Redmond CK et al. Endometrial cancer in tamoxifen-treated breast cancer patients: findings from the National Surgical Adjuvant Breast and Bowel Project (NSABP) B-14. *J Natl Cancer Inst* 1994;86:527–37.

Gøtzsche PC, Nielsen M. Screening for breast cancer with mammography. *Cochrane Database Syst Rev* 2009, issue 4. CD001877. www.thecochranelibrary.com

Howell A, Cuzick J, Baum M et al.; ATAC Trialists' Group. Results of the ATAC (Arimidex, Tamoxifen, Alone or in Combination) trial after completion of 5 years' adjuvant treatment for breast cancer. *Lancet* 2005;365:60–2.

Land SR, Wickerham DL, Costantino JP et al. Patient-reported symptoms and quality of life during treatment with tamoxifen or raloxifene for breast cancer prevention: The NSABP study of tamoxifen and raloxifene (STAR) P-2 Trial. *JAMA* 2006;295:2742–51.

Vaidya JS Women undergoing screening mammography experience a higher incidence of invasive breast cancer, without a corresponding reduction in symptomatic breast cancer. *BMJ Rapid Response* 20 July 2009. Available from www.bmj.com/cgi/eletters/339/jul09_1/b2587#217188, last accessed 1 Feb 2010.

Vogel VG, Costantino JP, Wickerham DL et al. for the National Surgical Adjuvant Breast and Bowel Project (NSABP). Effects of tamoxifen vs raloxifene on the risk of developing invasive breast cancer and other disease outcomes: The NSABP study of tamoxifen and raloxifene (STAR) P-2 Trial. *JAMA* 2006;295:2727–41.

3 Pathophysiology

The biological enigma

Breast cancer is an enigmatic disease. Although it is possible to make broad generalizations about risk, natural history and clinical pattern, the future for any individual woman (and the occasional man) who develops breast cancer is highly unpredictable. Consider the following observations.

- The risk of breast cancer begins at puberty and rises slowly until the perimenopausal years, when it increases dramatically, eventually leveling off at about the age of 75 years. Women who do not achieve menses seldom get breast cancer. The lifetime exposure to menstrual cycles, and particularly age at onset of menses, is one of the more important non-genetic risk factors.
- Breast cancer stage appears to be a biological property of the tumor rather than simply an expression of anatomic spread. The natural history of breast cancer is determined by the stage at diagnosis; thus, the risk of recurrence of a stage II tumor is inherently higher than that of a stage I tumor. However, irrespective of grade or stage, the risk of recurrence peaks at about 3 years, then flattens for a few years, with a second peak appearing between 7 and 10 years, before settling down to a constant hazard for the rest of the patient's life (breast cancers detected early by mammography may prove to be an exception). Puzzlingly, the stage only changes the height of the peaks rather than the timing after surgery, which remains constant.
- Although highly aggressive surgical procedures are no better than limited excision for local and systemic management of breast cancer, there is a clear link between local control and overall survival. A meta-analysis of randomized trials found that for every four local recurrences at 5 years prevented by better local treatment, one life is saved at 15 years. A recent elegant, albeit retrospective, analysis of these data suggests that this ratio of 4:1 may not be the same across various risk levels; the ratio reduces to nearly 1:1 for cancers with a good prognosis and increases to 1:infinity when the prognosis is poor.

This means that, for high-risk cancers, any improvement in local control may not change survival, while for cancers with a good prognosis, local control is very important. It appears that, when the prognosis is good, it is important to avoid local recurrence to prevent a secondary wave of metastatic growth either directly or as a result of its surgical diagnosis and treatment. It is important to remember that these data do not include any patients in whom the cancers were detected by screening, which may behave paradoxically, yielding a U-shaped curve.
- When breast cancer recurs, it can show a variety of presentations, depending on the time to relapse and the site of tissue recurrence. For example, the longer the disease-free interval, the better the prognosis and the more likely the tumor is to be estrogen-receptor positive or progesterone-receptor positive and to have metastasized to bone. (It is not known why metastasis to bone is associated with a better prognosis; it is most likely that bone metastasis causes less disturbance of the systemic physiology than lung or liver metastasis.)
- The anatomic distribution of the disease shows several curious clusters. In some cases, the tumor may be locally aggressive (particularly on the chest wall) and refractory to therapy, yet show little propensity to wider dissemination until much later. Bony metastases can wax and wane for years. Occasionally, the disease is explosive in both time and distribution, mimicking an infectious process. Histopathologically, the outcome cannot be predicted with certainty from the original tissue.
- Hormone manipulation is more effective in postmenopausal women than in younger women. For cytotoxic therapies, however, the opposite is true.

Breast biology

To appreciate the significance of the observations outlined above, it is helpful to consider the development of the human breast and breast cancer as a biological process.

The breast is an epithelial organ that develops in the embryo from the ectodermal primitive milk streak, or 'galactic band'. This ridge of tissue extends from the axilla to the groin, and is responsible for the supernumerary breasts occasionally seen in humans, and familiar in other mammalian species. The breast parenchyma is thought to develop from sweat glands, and is independent of hormonal influence during this early stage. By the third trimester of pregnancy, placental sex hormones enter the fetal circulation and induce canalization of early branched epithelial tissues. The 'witch's milk' that may occur in neonates of both sexes is secreted from these early glands.

The breast then remains relatively quiescent until puberty when, under the influence of hypothalamic gonadotropin-releasing hormones, primordial ovarian follicles mature and produce estrogens that stimulate the growth and maturation of breast and other sensitive tissues. With the onset of ovulatory menstrual cycles, the breast begins a period of cyclic stimulation and regression that continues until interrupted by pregnancy, the menopause or certain pharmacological or other intervention, such as intensive physical training.

Malignant change. It is, perhaps, a truism to suggest that breast cancer is the result of a subtle imbalance in the complex regulatory cycles to which breast tissue is exposed. Sex hormones, epidermal growth factors and other agents that influence normal growth and function do so by up- and downregulating genetic pathways, leading to cell proliferation and regression. The induction and promotion of breast cancer is a multifactorial and multistep process, in which a series of defenses must be overcome over a period of time, though not necessarily in a rigidly defined order. As this process develops from an early genetic predisposition, each defect in the regulatory system contributes to a cascade. In time, and in the face of numerous external stimuli, the family of defects expands, eventually leading to cellular immortalization and the molecular expression of the drivers of the classic malignant triad of growth, invasion and metastasis (Figure 3.1).

The subtle dividing line between benign and malignant changes is seen in ductal carcinoma in situ. There is now evidence that, in this situation, tumor sensitivity to growth hormones is increased, but the tumor lacks the abnormal ability to traverse the basement membrane, and thus may reach a considerable size yet remain localized. The subsequent emergence of the ability of the tumor to cross the basement

Pathophysiology

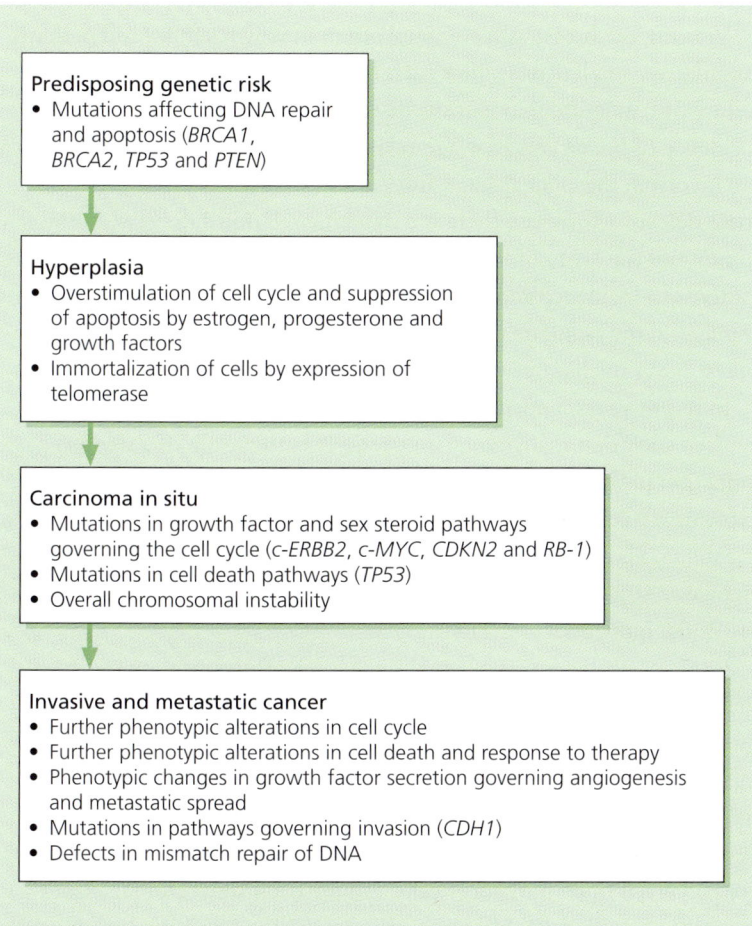

Figure 3.1 The genetic and phenotypic changes in mammary epithelial cells associated with the onset and progression of breast cancer.

membrane, apparently characterized by the production of specific gene products such as hyaluronidase, heralds invasion and increased risk of systemic disease. It is likely that each step in the triad of growth, invasion and metastasis is controlled by specific proteins secreted by the tumor or surrounding tissue. Thus, while the tissues from different patients may have the same histopathological appearance, the genetic and metabolic machinery will differ. The mixture of defects involved is likely to determine the clinical pattern of the disease.

Viewing the breast as a complex organ in which subtle, and perhaps cumulative, small defects after each menstrual cycle lead to an overall failure of regulation may put the disease process into context. The incidence of breast cancer is age-related perhaps because multiple defects are involved; the clinical stage and pattern of disease are functions of these defects. Moreover, there is a dynamic relationship between the tumor and the host, and thus the defects are themselves in constant flux. Patterns of incidence and recurrence seem to parallel known major changes in the regulatory milieu, such as the menopause and possibly other, as yet uncharacterized, events.

In recent years, understanding at the molecular and tissue levels has evolved such that malignancy is now seen as the result of a multistep induction process that never reaches an end point. It is a constantly evolving dynamic in which communities of cells lose their organizational discipline. Spontaneous and internally and externally driven genetic changes result in altered regulatory processes governing the day-to-day life of the individual cell (Figure 3.2).

Cancer cells were previously thought to be truly autonomous from their surroundings, but this is now known to be untrue. Cancer cells interact intensely with their surroundings; it is the signaling that is misguided. Paradoxically, cancer cells are often overly sensitive to otherwise appropriate stimuli. Moreover, cancer as a process extends beyond the cancer cell. The real action is at the interface between what are perceived to be the cancer cells and the ostensibly normal tissues adjacent to those cells. More recently, heritable epigenetic mechanisms have suggested explanations to some apparent paradoxes of the natural history of cancer.

More than 95% of breast cancers are epithelial tumors, arising from either the milk-producing glands (lobular carcinomas) or the draining ducts (ductal carcinomas). As an endocrine-related tumor, breast cancer shares with prostate, thyroid and other rarer epithelial malignancies an enigmatic, time-variable history quite distinct from other common epithelial tumors, such as those derived from the colon and lung. The patterns of long disease-free intervals followed by cyclic recurrence and remission are characteristic of these endocrine-related epithelial malignancies. The natural history of colon cancer, viewed from a

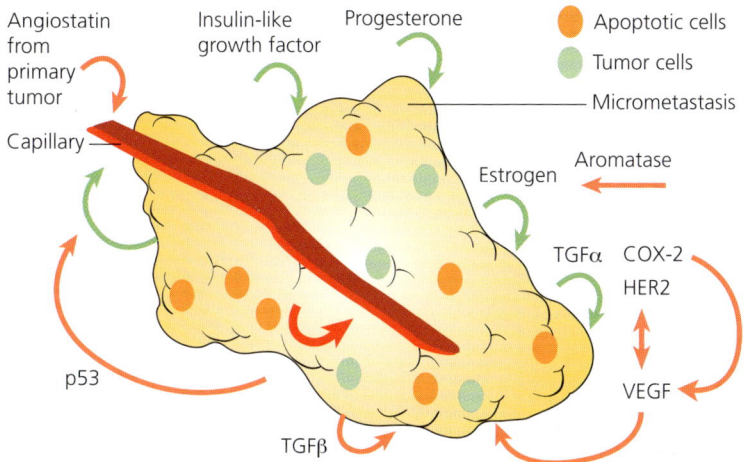

Figure 3.2 A schematic illustration of a hypothetical micrometastasis. The tumor is in a state of dynamic equilibrium as a result of its microenvironment; the 'soup' of cytokines in this environment balance angiogenesis, epithelial proliferation and apoptosis. Surgery may unbalance this equilibrium and 'kick-start' active growth, leading to the first peak in the incidence of clinically obvious secondary tumors within 2 years.

population perspective, has a flat tail of long-term survivors, apparently cured. Breast cancer is fundamentally different (Figure 3.3). The survival curve never flattens. The risk of recurrence, on a proportionate basis, remains constant for life and is determined by the initial stage of the tumor. Moreover, there have been observations of periods of somewhat increased recurrence risk 2–3 years after diagnosis. All of this suggests a very subtle regulatory process that has both spontaneous and therapy-associated perturbations. This has caused renewed controversy in the clinical and research literature about whether some or all of the benefits of adjuvant chemotherapy really reflect hormonal manipulation by another means, and whether the act of surgery 'kick-starts' the dormant metastases by inducing angiogenesis.

The current treatment guidelines presented in *Fast Facts: Breast Cancer* have been derived from a classic model of the disease, which is now evolving rapidly. As breast cancer is more fully understood as a

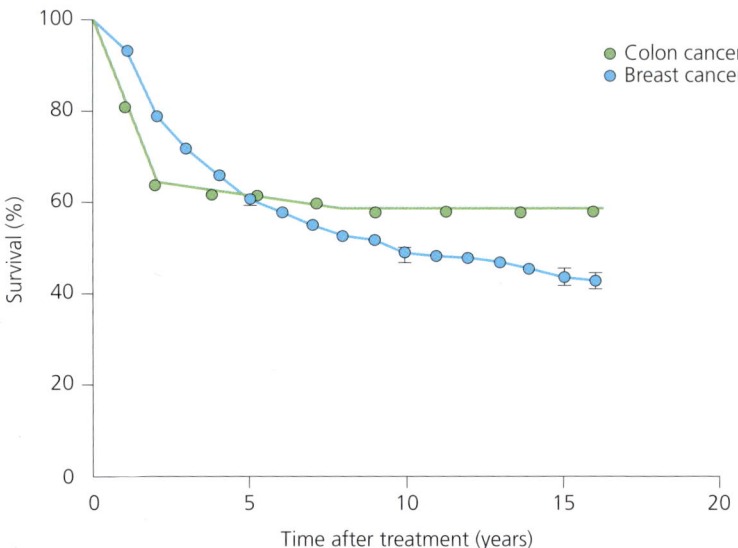

Figure 3.3 Comparison of survival in breast and colon cancer. In colon cancer, there is a flat tail on the survival curve after about 5 years and, in the absence of a second malignancy, these patients can be considered 'cured'. The breast cancer curve, however, does not exhibit such a tail. This biological difference underlies current treatment strategies and also offers insights into why the benefits of breast cancer interventions are likely to take longer to ascertain than those for colon cancer.

systemic regulatory disease with events at the time of surgery critical for outcome, treatment strategies will change, and perhaps the enigma will begin to dissipate.

Structure of the breast and surrounding tissues

The breast is composed of glandular and adipose tissue in varying proportions. The glandular tissue consists of 15–20 lobes containing numerous lobules, linked by ductules (Figure 3.4). The ductules combine to form the lactiferous ducts, which open into the lactiferous sinuses and empty through the nipple. The breast is enclosed in two layers of fibrous tissue connected by Cooper's ligaments: a superficial layer, and a thicker deep layer overlying the chest muscles.

Pathophysiology

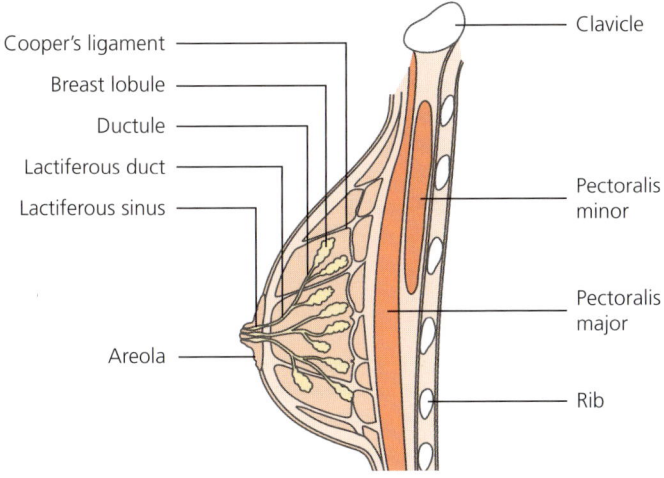

Figure 3.4 Structure of the normal breast.

The blood supply to the breast has two main components. The outer region of the breast is supplied by branches of the axillary artery, whereas the inner region is supplied by arteries arising from the internal mammary artery. Similarly, lymph from the outer region drains into the axillary lymph nodes, while lymph from the inner region is drained via the lymph nodes associated with the internal mammary artery.

The lymphatics of the breast tissue converge in the subareolar plexus of Sappy, which is convenient when performing a sentinel node biopsy (see pages 73–4).

Benign breast disease

Although a lump in the breast is the first symptom in 80–90% of cases of breast cancer, about 80% of breast lumps are due to benign breast disease (Table 3.1). Benign breast disease affects up to 30% of women; fibroadenomas and diffuse nodularity are most common in young women (< 30 years of age), whereas cysts are more common over the age of 40 years (Figure 3.5). Of note, dimpling of the skin is an almost pathognomic sign of cancer, being caused by the contracture of Cooper's ligaments by cicatrisation.

TABLE 3.1

Classification of benign breast disease

Benign neoplasia
- Fibroadenoma
- Lipoma
- Hamartoma
- Pseudoangiomatous stromal hyperplasia
- Duct papilloma
- Skin lesion

Dysplasia
- Abnormality of normal development and involution (nodularity)
- Solitary cyst
- Epithelial hyperplasia/atypia

Trauma
- Hematoma
- Fat necrosis

Inflammatory disease
- Puerperal abscess
- Periductal (plasma cell) mastitis
- Tuberculosis
- Diabetic mastopathy

Developmental
- Supernumerary breast
- Absent breast
- Asymmetrical breast development

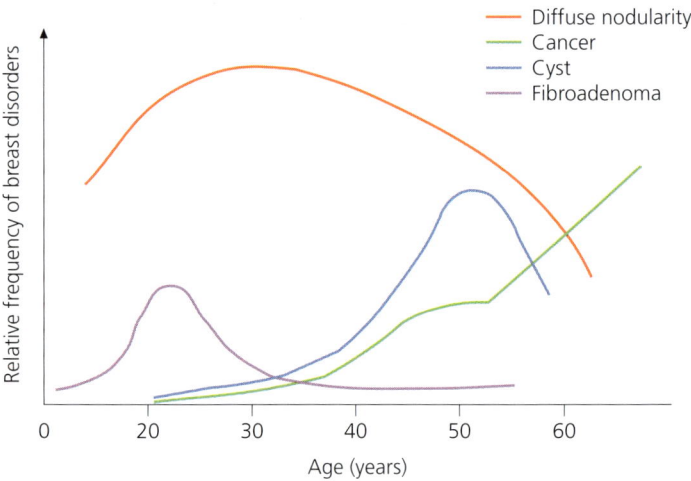

Figure 3.5 Fibroadenomas and diffuse nodularity are most common in women below 30 years of age. By contrast, benign cysts and breast cancer become more common after the age of 40 years.

Solitary cysts are among the most common benign breast tumors in women aged 35–55 years. They can be diagnosed and treated by needle aspiration of the cyst contents.

Fibroadenomas account for 13% of all breast tumors and are most common in women below 30 years of age, in whom they account for 60% of palpable lumps. Fewer than 10% of fibroadenomas increase in size and approximately one-third decrease in size or disappear. Fibroadenomas over 4 cm in diameter should be excised. Smaller tumors do not need to be excised in women under 35 years of age if the diagnosis has been confirmed by cytology. Excision is considered appropriate in older women to avoid the risk of overlooking breast cancer, unless the diagnosis has been confirmed by image-guided core biopsy.

Hamartoma are benign malformations of normal tissues of the breast that can either form a lump or an imaging abnormality. They are becoming diagnosed increasingly as many more biopsies are carried out in 'worried well' women.

Pseudoangiomatous stromal hyperplasia is another incidental finding considered to be a benign myofibroblastic proliferation of breast tissue. It may need local excision and should not be confused histologically with angiosarcoma.

Epithelial dysplasia may be a chance finding following biopsy of a 'lumpy breast'. The combination of epithelial hyperplasia and cellular atypia is termed atypical hyperplasia, and is a potentially premalignant condition; the 10-year risk of breast cancer if atypical hyperplasia is present is 8% for a woman without a first-degree relative with breast cancer, and 20–25% for a woman with an affected first-degree relative.

Breast cancer
Most malignant breast tumors originate in the epithelia of the terminal ducts and lobules; only a small number involve the stroma or soft tissues. The most common classification describes tumors on the basis

of their origins (ducts or lobules) and according to whether they are confined to their original site or have invaded surrounding tissues. There is emerging evidence that, like hematopoietic tissues, solid organs – including the breast – retain primordial stem cells. Regulatory defects in these cells have been identified, and may serve as the nidus of malignancy. If so, our diagnostic/treatment strategies will have to evolve.

Histologically, breast cancers are characterized by groups of abnormal cells in a matrix of normal fibrous tissue. The degree of differentiation can be expressed according to the Scarf, Bloom and Richardson scale, in which glandular formation, nuclear pleomorphism and frequency of mitoses are each scored from 1 to 3. Highly differentiated tumors (grade I, score 3–5) are associated with a better prognosis than poorly differentiated tumors (grade III, score 8–9).

Ductal carcinomas account for over 90% of breast cancers. They generally present as a hard, poorly defined lump. Involvement of the Cooper's ligaments and ducts leads to the characteristic dimpling and pitting of the skin, which can be quite far from the actual tumor, and nipple inversion (Figure 3.6). Dimpling of the skin is an early sign of cancer that is easily missed unless carefully sought and should not be confused with actual skin involvement, which is an indicator of a T4 tumor (see Staging of breast cancer, pages 40–3).

Lobular carcinomas account for approximately 8% of breast cancers. Such tumors may occur at several sites, either in the same breast or in both breasts. The physical signs and characteristics of lobular cancers

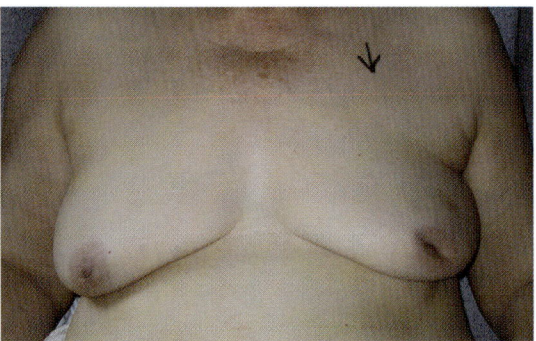

Figure 3.6 Clinical appearance of an invasive ductal carcinoma in the left breast of an elderly woman. Note the appearance of the nipple.

may be similar to those of ductal cancer. However, they are often hard to diagnose as their diffuse nature and relative radiolucency mean that they often do not show up on mammograms.

Phyllodes tumors (cystosarcoma phyllodes) are relatively rare stromal tumors. They do occasionally show cystic degeneration, but only very rarely exhibit the malignant features of a true sarcoma. Clinically and on imaging, they resemble fibroadenomas, although they are often larger than 2 cm in diameter. Microscopically the epithelial elements are normal, but the stromal areas show abnormal numbers of fibroblasts, some of which have a primitive morphology. They are subdivided into low grade (the majority) and high grade (about 5%). Low-grade tumors may be treated in the same manner as fibroadenomas, and high-grade tumors in the same way as sarcoma with radical excision. Like other stromal malignancies, these tumors tend to metastasize to the lung, but lymph-node metastases are not unknown. It is important to obtain a diagnosis by core biopsy before a fibroadenoma is excised, particularly in an older woman, so that a wider excision rather than enucleation can be performed at the outset.

Preinvasive lesions are referred to as ductal carcinomas or lobular carcinomas in situ. Lumps are seldom detectable, and most such tumors are detected by mammographic screening of the breast or as chance findings after a biopsy of a benign lesion. The proportion of in-situ carcinomas that progress to invasive disease is unknown, though postmortem studies suggest that it may be as low as 20%. The risk of invasive cancer is believed to be increased about eleven-fold in a woman in whom ductal carcinoma in situ is treated by removal of the affected area alone.

Natural history of breast cancer

At one extreme, women may present with massive involvement of the axillary nodes or even bone-marrow infiltration and a virtually undetectable primary tumor, and die of breast cancer before the primary disease is clinically apparent. At the other extreme, women may refuse treatment and live for 20–30 years with a slowly progressive cancer which, though it may present an unpleasant problem for the patient, seems to lack the capacity to metastasize and kill. Furthermore, following apparently successful treatment, women can relapse and die up to 20–30 years after the initial diagnosis. It is also curious that, irrespective of the disease-free interval between diagnosis and relapse, the subsequent behavior of the disease becomes predictable. No patients have been cured once distant relapse has been diagnosed, and the median expectation of survival is about 2 years, though the range is wide. Certainly, those patients with a longer disease-free interval are more likely to respond to endocrine treatments which, in rare cases, are associated with prolonged remission.

Of particular note is the aggressive nature of breast cancer in very young women; for those under the age of 34 years at diagnosis, fewer than half can be expected to survive 5 years, with most relapsing within the first 3 years after treatment. The prognostic significance of chest wall recurrence has also yet to be explained adequately. A patient may have a perfectly adequate mastectomy with wide margins of clearance on pathological assessment, but subsequently develop a crop of nodules on the chest wall, which are recurrent breast cancer, followed within a short interval by distant metastases, leading to death.

Nomenclature of breast cancer. The traditional adjective used to describe breast cancer – 'invasive' – is a tautology and is unnecessary. It is not used for other cancers: colon cancer is not called invasive colon cancer!

In the same vein, the term 'ductal' or 'lobular carinoma in situ' (DCIS and LCIS) should not be used to refer to preinvasive lesions. By definition they cannot spread and are cured by local excision (as long as there is no breach of the basement membrane so do not qualify as 'carcinoma'.

DIN (ductal intraepithelial neoplasia) similar to (CIN cervical intraepithelial neoplasia) would be the preferred name and would remove the unnecessary taboo of cancer when these lesions are diagnosed by mammographic screening.

Staging of breast cancer

Accurate clinical staging for breast cancer has always been considered essential as a guide to prognosis and treatment. It defines the limits of primary surgical approaches (see Chapter 5), and establishes the prognostic setting for radiation and systemic treatments. The original reason for this was the recognition, back in the early 1940s, that many of the locally advanced stages of the disease were incurable by radical surgery and often led to uncontrolled malignant ulceration across the chest wall. It is important to remember the clinical signs of breast cancer that would invalidate surgical attempts at cure, when initial referral to a medical oncologist would be more relevant (Table 3.2). Staging has also become important for selecting those patients who would most benefit from adjuvant systemic therapy (see Chapter 6), but these indices depend heavily on histological and biological variables. Thus anatomic mapping has become part of a broader staging strategy.

The currently used staging system is based on the clinical size and extent of invasion of the primary tumor (T), the clinical absence or presence of palpable axillary lymph nodes and evidence of their local invasion (N), together with the clinical and imaging evidence of distant metastases (M). This is known as the TNM classification (Table 3.3).

The principal measures used at present are invasion (a measure of invasive potential), nodal status (metastatic potential), tumor size (growth potential), histological grade (growth rate and regulatory

TABLE 3.2
Clinical signs precluding surgery

- Inflammatory changes throughout the breast
- Peau d'orange involving more than 30% of the breast surface area
- Ulceration of the skin (a relative contraindication; surgery may be technically possible for salvage)
- Fixation of the tumor to the underlying chest wall (fixation to muscle alone is a relative contraindication that can be judged clinically; surgery may be technically feasible for salvage)
- Fixation of the axillary lymph nodes to the chest wall or the neurovascular bundle supplying the arm
- Overt, distant metastatic disease, where the expectation of life is less than 2 years

TABLE 3.3
The tumor–nodes–metastases (TNM) classification of breast cancer

Tumor status

TX	Primary tumor cannot be assessed
T0	No evidence of primary tumor
Tis	Carcinoma in situ
T1	Tumor ≤ 2 cm
T1a	Tumor ≤ 0.5 cm
T1b	Tumor > 0.5 cm but < 1 cm
T1c	Tumor > 1 cm but < 2 cm
T2	Tumor > 2 cm but < 5 cm
T3	Tumor > 5 cm
T4	Tumor of any size with direct extension to the chest wall or skin
T4a	Extension to the chest wall
T4b	Edema (including peau d'orange), skin ulceration or satellite skin nodules confined to the same breast
T4c	Both T4a and T4b
T4d	Inflammatory carcinoma

Status of lymph nodes

NX	Regional lymph nodes cannot be assessed (e.g. removed previously)
N0	No regional lymph-node metastasis
N1	Metastasis to movable ipsilateral axillary nodes
nN2	Metastases in ipsilateral axillary lymph nodes fixed or matted, or in clinically apparent* ipsilateral internal mammary nodes in the absence of clinically evident axillary lymph node metastasis
nN2a	Metastasis in ipsilateral axillary lymph nodes fixed to one another (matted) or to other structures

CONTINUED

TABLE 3.3 (CONTINUED)

nN2b	Metastasis only in clinically apparent* ipsilateral internal mammary nodes and in the *absence* of clinically evident axillary lymph node metastasis
nN3	Metastasis in ipsilateral infraclavicular lymph node(s) with or without axillary lymph node involvement, or in clinically apparent* ipsilateral internal mammary lymph node(s) and in the *presence* of clinically evident axillary lymph node metastasis; or metastasis in ipsilateral supraclavicular lymph node(s) with or without axillary or internal mammary lymph node involvement
nN3a	Metastasis in ipsilateral infraclavicular lymph node(s)
nN3b	Metastasis in ipsilateral internal mammary lymph node(s) and axillary lymph node(s)
nN3c	Metastasis in ipsilateral supraclavicular lymph node(s)

Distant metastases

M0	No clinically apparent distant metastases
M1	Distant metastases obvious

*Clinically apparent is defined as detected by imaging studies (excluding lymphoscintigraphy) or by clinical examination or grossly visible pathologically.

potential) and hormone receptor status. In addition, a measure of overproduction of human epidermal growth factor receptor 2 is now becoming part of standard care. Oddly, most staging systems do not take into account any surrogate marker for growth rate of the primary tumor.

In addition to the classic clinical staging systems, more and more prognostic variables are being added, which may be mathematically subsumed into a global prognostic index. A well-known example of this is the Nottingham Prognostic Index (NPI; Table 3.4), which incorporates histological grade, tumor size and the extent of lymph-node infiltration. Although the NPI is widely used for assessing prognosis and guiding treatment, better and more sophisticated web-based tools are now available. Some of these have been well validated (e.g. Adjuvant! Online, www.adjuvantonline.com) while others are being tested (e.g. www.nemc.org/ibtr, www.cancer-math.net).

TABLE 3.4
The Nottingham Prognostic Index
The figure shows prognostic sub-groups based on the Index

Histological grade	Score

To determine the grade, add the scores for each component:
3–5 = grade I; 6–7 = grade II; 8–9 = grade III

Tubule formation

Majority of tumor (> 75%)	1
Moderate amount (10–75%)	2
Little or none (< 10%)	3

Nuclear size

Regular, uniform	1
Larger variation	2
Marked variation	3

Mitotic frequency — Depends on microscope field size

Nodal stage

Node sampling: low axillary, apical axillary and internal mammary nodes

Stage A

Tumor absent from all nodes sampled at all three sites	1

Stage B

Tumor in a low axillary node only (or) in an internal mammary node only (or) in three or fewer nodes in an axillary clearance	2

Stage C

Tumor in apical node (or) in low axillary node plus internal mammary nodes (or) in four or more nodes in axillary clearance	3

Nottingham Prognostic Index = (0.2 × size in cm) + grade + stage

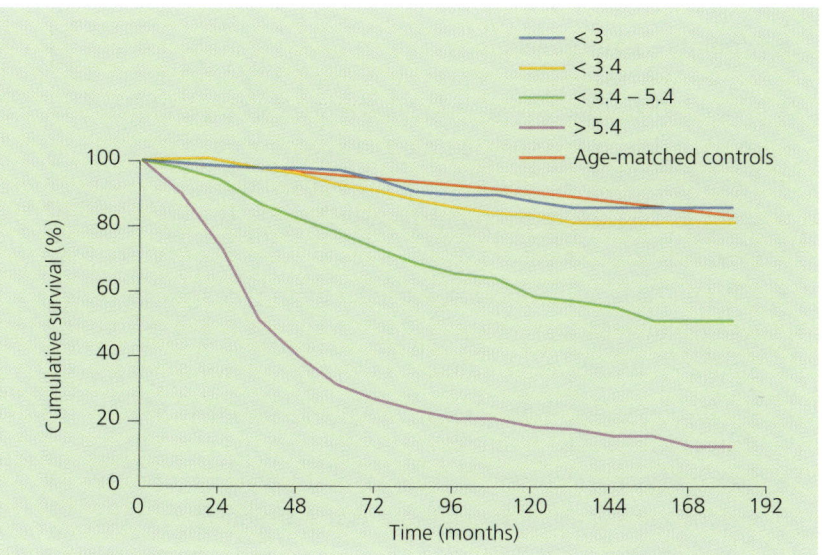

Prognostic factors

It is reasonable to describe the natural history of breast cancer in terms of growth, invasion and metastatic potential. These properties are genetically controlled through the production of specific proteins. They are probably also time-dependent, with a tendency to become less controllable, and they are affected by the local milieu. Current prognostic indicators are largely indirect measures of these properties, and achieve about 60% accuracy.

Gene array technology, which allows the genetic activity in different tissues to be characterized and compared, is now beginning to influence clinical medicine. Malignancies, particularly leukemias and lymphomas, are being classified by gene-expression patterns in addition to conventional light microscopy and flow cytometry. Patterns of gene expression appear to correlate with light-microscopic diagnosis. Moreover, data are accumulating to allow clinicians to estimate the risk of relapse, its likely pattern and its response to specific treatments with greater precision. The current challenge is to make the technique sufficiently robust and reproducible for wider use.

Key points – pathophysiology

- Breast cancer is becoming understood as a constantly evolving series of defects in cellular regulation and control.
- Growth, invasion and metastasis are related but distinct regulatory processes. The mix determines the clinical course in an individual patient.
- Most breast lumps are benign, especially those in women younger than 50 years of age.
- Staging of breast cancer, including examination of lymph nodes, is a prognosis-estimating procedure. It is not therapeutic other than in achieving local control.
- New evidence is emerging that the act of surgery itself, or even major trauma at a later stage, might induce angiogenesis at the site of latent/occult distant metastases.
- Gene array techniques are bringing modern molecular biology into the clinic.

Key references

Dixon JM. Hormone replacement therapy and the breast. *BMJ* 2001;323:1381–2.

Gnant M, Mlineritsch B, Schippinger W et al. Endocrine therapy plus zoledronic acid in premenopausal breast cancer. *N Engl J Med* 2009;360:679–91.

Hankinson SE, Willett WC, Colditz GA et al. Circulating concentrations of insulin-like growth factor-I and risk of breast cancer. *Lancet* 1998;351:1393–6.

Hedenfalk I, Duggan D, Chen Y et al. Gene-expression profiles in hereditary breast cancer. *N Engl J Med* 2001;344:539–48.

Huang, E, Cheng SH, Dressman H et al. Gene expression predictors of breast cancer outcomes. *Lancet* 2003;361:1590–6.

Kelsey JL, Bernstein L. Epidemiology and prevention of breast cancer. *Annu Rev Public Health* 1996;17:47–67.

Ntzani EE, Ioannidis JPA. Predictive ability of DNA microarrays for cancer outcomes and correlates: an empirical assessment. *Lancet* 2003;362:1439–44.

Peto R, Boreham J, Clarke M et al. UK and USA breast cancer deaths down 25% in year 2000 at ages 29–60 years. *Lancet* 2000;355:1822.

4 Diagnosis

Symptoms of breast cancer

Although a lump in the breast is the most common presenting symptom of breast cancer, a variety of other symptoms may be present (Table 4.1).

Lumps resulting from breast cancer are generally single, hard and painless, and may be irregular in shape. Fibroadenomas, however, may also appear as single, hard lumps. Typically, breast cancers are about 2 cm in diameter by the time they become large enough to be palpable. Approximately 60% arise in the upper outer quadrant of the breast, but any area of the breast can be affected.

Pain in the breast is seldom due to cancer. The most common cause is the normal periodic pain during the menstrual cycle (cyclic mastalgia). In many cases, it is due to costochondritis (Tietze's syndrome) and it is

TABLE 4.1

Symptoms that may indicate breast cancer

- Lump in the breast
- Dimpling of the skin of the breast
- Bleeding or discharge from the nipple
- Breast pain
- Changes in the size or shape of the breast
- Involution or inversion of the nipple
- Lump in the armpit
- Swelling of the arm (lymphedema)
- Ulceration of the skin
- Symptoms of secondary tumors, such as bony pain, loss of appetite, breathlessness and headache

possible that referred pain from this may explain many cases of non-cyclical mastalgia; the pathophysiology of Tietze's syndrome is poorly understood. However, pain does not exclude a cancer.

Bleeding from the nipple is a rare symptom of breast cancer; fewer than 3% of women report bleeding as a first symptom. The likelihood of cancer is increased if a lump is found on examination. In the absence of a lump, the most common cause of bleeding or bloodstained discharge is benign duct papilloma. In postmenopausal women, discharges from the nipple that are not bloodstained are usually due to duct ectasia. Discharges may also occur during early pregnancy, after breast-feeding, and during treatment with certain drugs, such as oral contraceptives, some antihypertensive agents and some antidepressants. Persistent discharge from a single duct in the nipple needs to investigated, especially if a dipstick is positive for blood. The usual method is microdochectomy (removal of a single duct), or in older women, total duct excision; the value of ductoscopy is being investigated.

Changes in size or shape of the breasts may also indicate breast cancer. The affected breast may increase in size or become pendulous; conversely, in advanced breast cancer the breast may shrink owing to loss of normal breast tissue and retraction because of cicatrization. The skin may dimple or pucker because of edema and infiltration of Cooper's ligaments, and the nipple may become inverted. The veins in the breast may become more prominent as the tumor enlarges.

Skin involvement. In advanced cases, the tumor may involve the skin, leading to ulceration (Figure 4.1). Blockage of the lymphatic circulation can cause lymphedema, resulting in swelling of the arm. Accumulation of fluid in the dermis, which maintains its thickness at the sites of sweat glands and hair follicles, causes the typical 'peau d'orange' (orange skin) appearance. This is a late sign of cancer (stage T4).

Lymph nodes. Occasionally, it is not possible to identify the primary tumor, and the only evidence of breast cancer is enlarged lymph nodes.

Diagnosis

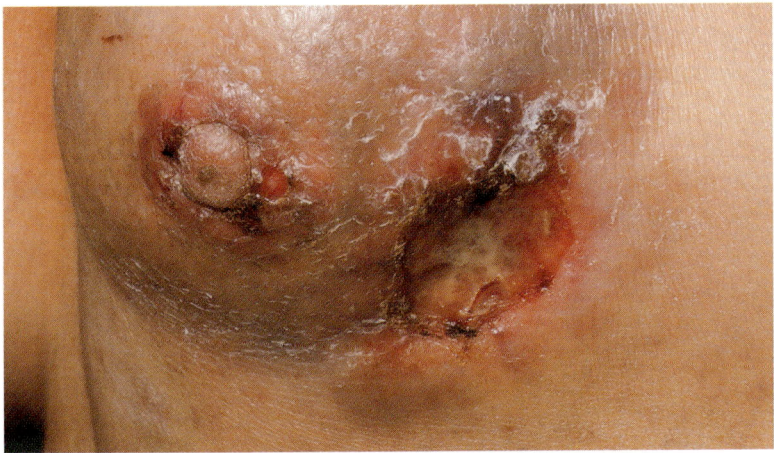

Figure 4.1 Ulcerating local recurrence in the breast and nipple after wide local excision and radiotherapy some years before.

However, a few women find the axillary lump first and can feel the breast lump only after the doctor shows it to them.

Metastatic breast cancer can cause a variety of symptoms, including bone pain, breathlessness, nausea and jaundice. It is, however, rare for a woman to present with metastatic disease.

When to refer?

Breast symptoms that require referral to a specialist physician/surgeon or clinic are summarized in Table 4.2. The following patient groups can be managed, at least initially, by the primary care physician:

- young women with tender, lumpy breasts and older women with symmetrical nodularity provided that no localized abnormality is present or family history (Figure 4.2)
- women with minor or moderate breast pain who do not have a palpable lesion
- women of any age who have nipple discharge that is from one or more ducts, or is intermittent, and is neither bloodstained nor troublesome.

There is no single test or group of tests that provides perfect accuracy in the diagnosis of breast cancer. An 'index of suspicion' remains

TABLE 4.2

Symptoms requiring specialist referral

Lumps
- Any new discrete lump
- A new lump in pre-existing nodularity
- Asymmetrical nodularity persisting at review after menstruation
- Abscess
- Persistently refilling or recurrent cyst*
- Axillary or supraclavicular nodes

Pain
- Associated with a lump
- Intractable pain not responding to reassurance, simple measures such as wearing a well-fitting bra, or common drugs
- Persistent unilateral pain in postmenopausal women

Nipple discharge
- All women aged over 50 years
- Women aged below 50 years with:
  - bilateral discharge sufficient to stain clothes
  - bloodstained discharge
  - persistent discharge from a single duct

Nipple retraction or distortion, or nipple eczema

Change in skin contour

Family history
- A request from a woman with a strong family history of breast cancer (such patients should be referred to a family cancer genetics clinic where possible)

*Aspiration is acceptable if the patient has recurrent multiple cysts.

the paramount principle. A suspicious mass with negative mammographic findings warrants biopsy. Negative biopsy findings in such a patient should be reviewed for anatomical and histopathological accuracy.

Diagnosis

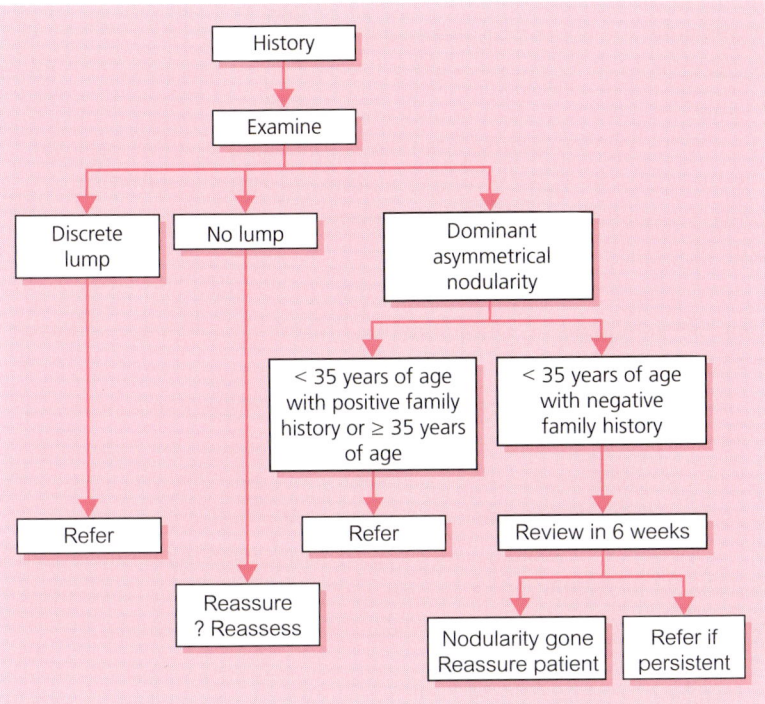

Figure 4.2 Guidelines for the management of patients with breast lumps.

Triple assessment

Triple assessment, which comprises clinical examination, imaging investigations and pathological evaluation, will enable a confident diagnosis in 95% of patients with suspected breast cancer.

History. A thorough history is crucial and its importance cannot be overemphasized; for example, a history of regular ibuprofen use in a young girl suggested a diagnosis of fibromatosis for a lump that otherwise mimicked breast cancer. A standard 'breast history' includes:
- a history of the presenting complaint, such as duration, associated pain (a cyst is often painful and tender at the outset), discharge, change in size; a menstrual, obstetric and gynecologic history
- the family history of breast and ovarian cancer
- a drug history including use of oral contraceptives and hormone replacement therapy

- previous and concurrent diseases and surgery
- allergies
- smoking.

A social history and an understanding of the family and occupational circumstances are also important, because the treatment of breast cancer can span several months and psychological support needs to be individualized.

Clinical examination is an essential first step in the diagnosis of breast cancer. A gentle examination is the key to success.

The patient should be examined sitting up with her hands in three positions: by her sides, above her head and pressing on her hips. This can reveal nipple retraction, or asymmetry and dimpling of the overlying skin. Sometimes the dimpling becomes apparent only when the patient bends forwards completely. Dimpling is often present in breast cancer and should be recognized as an early (rather than late) sign. It occurs because of contracture of the ligaments of Cooper that traverse the breast and attach to the dermis.

The patient should then be asked to lie in a semi-recumbent position and the breasts examined quadrant by quadrant with the flat of a (warm) hand; lubricating the skin often makes this examination more sensitive. This procedure can distinguish between a distinct lump and coarse nodular tissue, which is a common feature of benign dysplasia. The axillary nodes and supra- and infraclavicular nodes are then examined by palpation under the arms, above and below the collarbone, and from the front and the back of the patient.

Women who present with nipple discharge should be asked to massage the subareolar area to provoke secretion. The color and site of discharge should be noted and tested for presence of blood. Discharge from a single duct is usually due to a duct papilloma. The likelihood of finding carcinoma is about 1%.

Imaging. Both mammography and ultrasonography have important roles in the diagnosis of breast cancer, but the use of other modalities, such as magnetic resonance and infrared imaging, is being developed.

Mammography has a diagnostic accuracy of over 95% for clinically detectable tumors, and approximately 50% for subclinical cancers; this reduces to about 35% if cancers found only on whole organ analysis of mastectomy specimens are included. The technique can provide single oblique views of each breast, or both lateral and craniocaudal views. However, because it involves compressing the breast between two plates, the procedure can be uncomfortable.

Although mammography contributes little to the management of a patient with a discrete palpable lump, in whom the diagnosis should be based on cytology and histology if appropriate, it does have an important role in specific situations.

- Mammography may increase the likelihood of detecting a relatively small cancer in patients whose breasts have a coarse nodular texture.
- The technique can be used to locate the cancer accurately for excision biopsy (Figure 4.3).
- In women with a palpable lump, mammography may reveal an impalpable lump in the same or opposite breast. It should therefore be a prerequisite before conservative breast surgery is undertaken.
- Women who have undergone mastectomy for breast cancer are at increased risk of developing cancer in the remaining breast, and regular mammography may be useful for monitoring.

Mammography is also the most common method for localizing impalpable tumors prior to surgery (see Figure 4.6).

It should be remembered that mammography is particularly insensitive when the breasts are radiographically dense.

Ultrasonography has now become part of the standard evaluation of clinical abnormalities in the breast.

- Ultrasound has a specificity of over 95% in distinguishing a solid mass from a cystic mass (Figure 4.4); the diagnosis can then be confirmed and treated (in the case of a simple cyst) by needle aspiration. Improvements in technology have also increased both the sensitivity and specificity of ultrasound in the diagnosis of solid breast lumps. Benign lumps are well circumscribed with no acoustic shadow or isodense echoes, whereas malignant lumps have irregular outlines, are poorly defined and are variable in density or have echoes suggestive of microcalcifications.

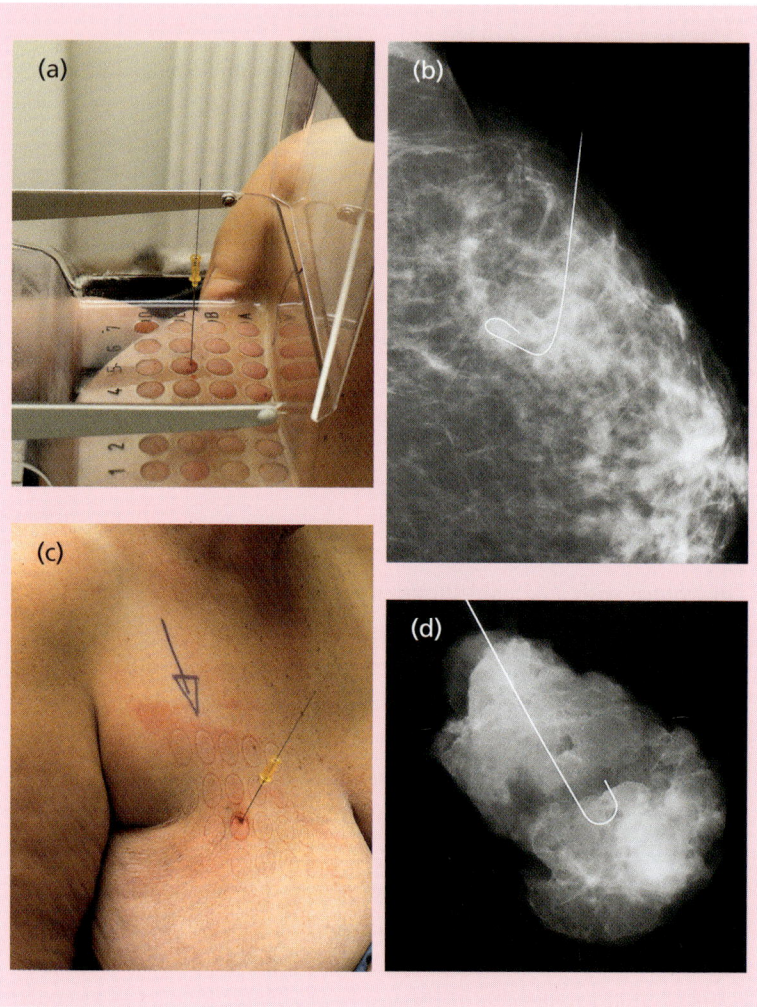

Figure 4.3 Mammography can be used to locate the tumor accurately before open biopsy. (a) Under local anesthesia, the breast is compressed in the mammogram unit and a needle inserted through a grid overlying the suspected tumor location. (b) Craniocaudal and oblique mammograms are then taken to ensure that the needle is lying close to the tumor. (c) The patient is next taken to the operating theater with the needle in situ. (d) The needle and the suspected tumor are excised and sent for radiological examination to confirm that the suspicious area has been removed before the wound is closed.

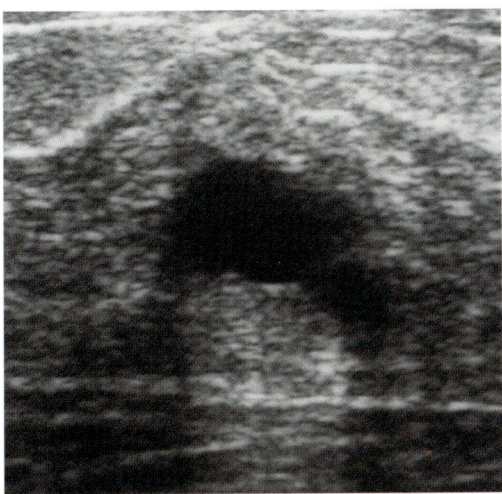

Figure 4.4 Simple cyst shown on ultrasound scan. Note the smooth margins, hypoechoic center and posterior acoustic enhancement.

- Distinguishing discrete lumps from areas of nodularity in a relatively young woman can be difficult. Ultrasound can provide reassurance if it fails to detect any localized abnormality.
- Ultrasound is used routinely to guide fine-needle aspiration cytology and to localize subclinical lesions with needles prior to excision biopsy.
- The use of ultrasound with enhanced color Doppler assessment of blood flow is now the primary tool for assessment of axillary metastases. In addition to detecting masses, it can detect increased vascularity, which can indicate lymph-node involvement. Assessment of the axilla is now part of the standard procedure that includes either guided cytology or core biopsy of a suspicious lymph node; if malignancy is found, sentinel node biopsy is unnecessary and axillary clearance can be performed at the time of the first operation.
- Enhanced color Doppler ultrasound scanning of the breast postoperatively is likely to improve the early diagnosis of local recurrence, which is otherwise difficult to achieve because of surgical scarring and the effects of radiotherapy.

Magnetic resonance. After the initial explosion of interest in magnetic resonance imaging (MRI) of the breast, concerns about its overuse are now being raised. Most importantly, the possibility that MRI may reduce either the necessity for re-operation or the likelihood of recurrence has not been fulfilled. It does, however, delay surgery and detect additional lesions that can prompt more extensive surgery, which has been shown to be of no benefit. However, the expense is now less of an issue, as the cost of the additional MRI breast coil is a fraction of the total cost of an MRI machine.

MRI, which is based on the nuclear spin of molecules within a powerful magnetic field, is free of the hazards of conventional X-ray imaging. It produces remarkable digitized images that allow three-dimensional reconstruction of the breast (Figure 4.5). Furthermore, injection of a contrast agent enables the vascularity of the lesion of interest to be visualized either as a dynamic function of uptake or as a static image (Figure 4.5b). However, an experienced radiological and surgical team is needed to interpret the images appropriately.

MRI may aid the diagnosis and management of breast cancer in certain clinical situations. However, in the authors' opinion, caution should be exercised to avoid ascribing undue importance to 'latent' lesions at a distance from the dominant primary, which persuades many surgeons to recommend a mastectomy. This clearly ignores evidence from the clinical trials of the past, which point to the safety of breast-conserving techniques. Large series have found that patients who underwent breast-conserving surgery after a preoperative MRI (therefore excluding those in whom additional lesions were found) have the same outcome as those who did not have a preoperative MRI evaluation, suggesting that the lesions found on MRI may never have progressed to a clinical tumor. The recently published Comparative

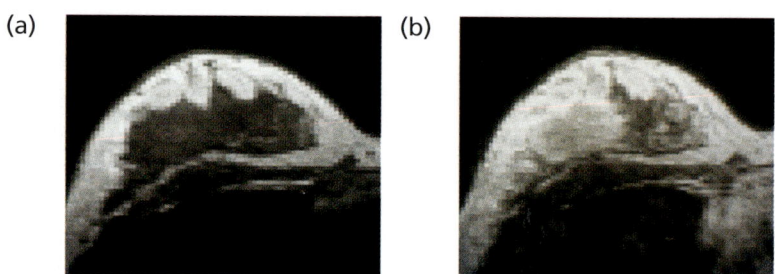

Figure 4.5 Typical appearance of breast cancer on magnetic resonance imaging (a) before and (b) after the injection of an enhancing agent. Reproduced courtesy of Mr Michael Douek.

Effectiveness of MRI in Breast Cancer (COMICE) trial that randomized women to either receive or not receive a preoperative MRI, found that MRI does not reduce re-operation rates (even with lobular cancers), but increases the mastectomy rates (7% vs 1%). No difference in local recurrence was found, although we need to await longer-term results before we dispense with the use of preoperative MRI.

A high-impact study found that additional cancers found on MRI in the contralateral breast may have prompted an increase in contralateral mastectomy rates, especially in the USA. After MRI and magnetic-resonance-guided biopsy of the contralateral breast, some women are increasingly opting for a contralateral prophylactic mastectomy, even if the biopsy is benign. This appears to be more likely if the woman is having a reconstruction. There is no evidence that such a drastic measure saves lives, and the availability of a good reconstruction service should not be an excuse for mastectomy of either the breast with the primary tumor or the contralateral side, even if lobular carcinoma is present.

Pathology. If a discrete lump is present, and clinical examination and ultrasound suggests that it is a cyst, it can be aspirated with a 10/20-mL syringe and venipuncture (blue hub) needle. Aspiration of non-bloody fluid confirms the diagnosis of a benign cyst and the fluid need not be sent for further examination. Such aspiration will provide immediate relief and reassurance. Biochemical examination of the fluid, albeit interesting, has no clinical relevance; and cytological examination can yield non-specific changes that can sometimes lead to unnecessary anxiety.

A bloodstained aspirate may indicate the presence of an intracystic cancer requiring open biopsy (see page 59). If the lump is solid, fine-needle aspiration can be used to obtain cells for cytological examination which, in some centers, can be completed within 30 minutes.

Fine-needle aspiration cytology (FNAC) was popularized in Sweden decades ago and has been widely adopted in the rest of Europe, though it is less commonly used in the USA. The technique is simple, and a skilled operator can usually produce an adequate sample from very small tumors by inserting the needle either into a clinically palpable lump or stereotactically under radiological or ultrasound control. The aspirate is immediately smeared on a series of slides and stained for conventional microscopic examination (Figure 4.6).

Experienced cytopathologists can diagnose breast cancer with almost 100% specificity. The sensitivity (i.e. false-negative rate) depends to a large extent on the operating skills of the clinician taking the sample and the experience of the cytologist. In many centers around the world where cytopathology results have been audited, surgeons are happy to carry out definitive cancer surgery on this result alone. However, the trend is changing worldwide, perhaps prompted by the few false-negative results that may have delayed a cancer diagnosis.

Biopsy. If cytological examination of cells obtained by FNAC is equivocal or not concordant with clinical or radiological features, especially in women over a certain age (i.e. > 35 years), a core biopsy should be obtained using an automatic core biopsy needle (widely available and, in many cases, disposable) under local anesthesia. Histological examination of the sample can then be used to confirm the cancer diagnosis.

An image-guided core biopsy with examination of at least four core specimens is recommended before a lump is confirmed as benign. The clinical and imaging findings should also be concordant. Modern core-cut biopsy techniques are considered the 'standard of care', particularly for lesions detected on screening.

Mammotome. A mammotome is a device that can sample a large amount of tissue using a specialized needle apparatus that uses a

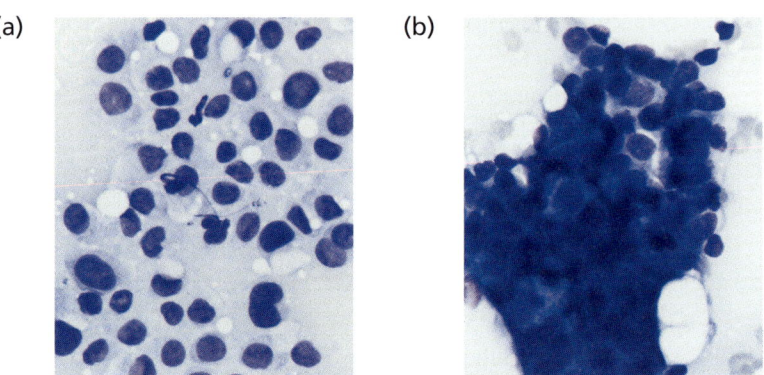

Figure 4.6 Examples of (a) malignant and (b) benign cytology.

vacuum to suck breast tissue towards the needle receptacle. As there is less sampling error, the false-negative rate is reduced to a very low level. It is increasingly being used, especially for lesions detected by screening. If the lesion is particularly small, it is prudent for the radiologist to insert a tiny radio-opaque clip at the site of the lesion, as it may be difficult to localize later if cancer is diagnosed.

Open biopsy involves the removal of the entire lump under general anesthesia. This procedure is associated with significant morbidity; approximately 20% of patients develop a further lump under the scar, or experience pain at the biopsy site. Thus, it should only be performed in patients who have been fully investigated by FNAC, mammography and core biopsy, and in whom the diagnosis still remains equivocal.

Metastatic spread

If the tumor is large and there is extensive lymph-node involvement, preoperative staging is prudent. This typically involves chest and abdominal computed tomography, and a bone scan, though a chest radiograph and ultrasound of the abdomen are also considered adequate. MRI and positron emission tomography are sometimes used for staging indeterminate lesions.

It should be emphasized that routine staging for metastatic spread in early breast cancer, especially when detected by screening or a node-negative T1 tumor is present, is not advisable as the yield is less than 4%. The investigations can result in equivocal results that are clinically irrelevant, but can delay the definitive treatment and provoke considerable anxiety.

Breast screening and breast awareness

The aim of screening for breast cancer is to reduce mortality by detecting tumors before they have spread beyond the breast. Since over 90% of breast cancers are first detected by the woman herself, the rationale for regular self-examination is to increase the likelihood of detecting a tumor as early as possible.

Screening. There is evidence that screening for breast cancer by regular mammography can reduce the risk of mortality from breast cancer by

20–30% in certain groups. Significant benefits are, however, seen only in women over the age of 50 years. In trials in Sweden, for example, mortality during 12 years of follow-up was reduced by 29% in women over 50 years of age, compared with only 13% in younger women. Furthermore, the reduction in younger women was not statistically significant, and was delayed by at least 8 years. There is, therefore, no evidence to support regular screening in women under 50 years of age. This is an ongoing controversy. The current medical consensus suggests that the relative risk reduction achieved by regular screening mammography in the 50–65-year-old age group is about 18%. The absolute risk reduction is much smaller, because the background risk of dying from breast cancer is about 3% in the general population.

It is worth noting that consumer advocacy groups also hold this viewpoint. The National Breast Cancer Coalition (NBCC) in the USA states: 'Women deserve to know the truth – and the truth is that there is no evidence of a mortality reduction in women under the age of 50 and the evidence for women over the age of 50 is currently unclear. Broad public health recommendations should only be made when it is clear that the potential benefits of the recommended intervention will outweigh the potential harms. NBCC believes that women are capable of educating themselves so that they can make their own individual decisions about screening.'

Screening programs for breast cancer are associated with a number of problems.

- Only about 70–80% of women accept mammography. It is much lower in some areas.
- Of all the cancers diagnosed, over 50% are diagnosed between screening mammograms.
- It is possible that a woman who is reassured by a negative result might ignore changes in her breasts between mammograms. Since 20–30% of breast cancers are not detected by mammography, some tumors could, therefore, be missed.
- False-positive results are obtained in about 1% of mammograms. Such results could generate unnecessary anxiety, particularly if further investigations are undertaken.

- For every breast cancer detected, a substantial number of women will undergo biopsies or surgery for benign breast disease, with attendant morbidity.
- Although the total dose of radiation received during mammography is low (< 1.5 mGy), it has been suggested that repeated exposure could increase the risk of breast cancer. This risk is, however, low. It has been estimated that screening 2 million women over 50 years of age by a single mammogram would result in one extra case of breast cancer each year after 10 years; by contrast, the normal incidence of breast cancer in women over 60 years of age is approximately 2000 cases/million.
- Small breast cancers detected by mammography may be biologically different from those detected clinically. Approximately 20% of cancers detected by mammography are carcinomas in situ, of which some would never progress to invasive disease if left undetected, and the optimal treatment for such tumors is unknown. If these cancers are treated in the same way as invasive cancers, some women may undergo unnecessarily extensive surgery. Conversely, in other women, delaying treatment of asymptomatic disease may ultimately compromise the chance of cure. Furthermore, there is good evidence (see Jørgensen and Gøtzsche, 2009, and www.bmj.com/cgi/eletters/339/jul09_1/b2587#217188) that screening leads to overdiagnosis. Many invasive cancers detected by screening would never have progressed to clinical disease.
- For every 2000 women screened for 10 years, 44 (vs 34 if not screened) cancers would be diagnosed, and there would be one fewer death.
- The optimum interval between mammograms has not been determined. The UK screening program currently recommends screening at 3-year intervals, but this is judged to be too long by some advocates of screening. Yet to shorten the interval would have major cost implications.
- Thus, although radiographic screening is the 'standard of care' in many places, it remains controversial.

The issue of risk and its importance when discussing screening with women is discussed on pages 21–2. One of the most important benefits of a screening programme is that it can raise the quality of investigation and complete multidisciplinary management of breast diseases to the highest level.

Breast self-examination. In the latter part of the 20th century, several large-scale programs were established to teach self-examination techniques and encourage women to examine their breasts each month. However, although this approach does appear to lead to the detection of smaller tumors, there is no evidence that it improves long-term survival. Indeed, two large-scale randomized controlled trials performed in St Petersburg and China found no difference in breast cancer mortality rates between women trained in breast self-examination and a control group. In these trials, compliance with the instructions was very high and could not be the reason for the absence of benefit. An adverse effect of training in self-examination was the disproportionate number of women presenting with lumpy breasts who were then subjected to futile biopsies. The self-examination approach also has a potential problem in that random biopsies among premenopausal women may disclose ductal carcinoma in situ or lobular carcinoma in situ, the natural history of which is unknown. Such findings may result in inappropriate radical surgery or, at the very least, a lifetime of uncertainty and anxiety for the patient.

In 2001, the Canadian Medical Association went one step further when it published new guidelines following a systematic review of the literature. As a public health measure, self-examination was relegated from category C (of no proven value) to category D (of proven harm)! This report, as expected, provoked storms of protest on both sides of the Atlantic. The controversy has deep roots. Part of the difficulty lies in the intuitive notion that detecting a tumor 'earlier' (i.e. when it is smaller) is necessarily better, but it is becoming apparent that not all breast cancers are the same, even if they appear so morphologically. Thus the disappointing results with early diagnostic attempts, including both imaging and self-examination, probably reflect our incomplete understanding of breast cancer as a process.

In the UK, emphasis was cleverly switched to 'breast awareness' rather than regular self-examination. In this approach, women are encouraged to become familiar with their breasts and to distinguish between normal cyclic fluctuations and abnormal changes for which medical advice should be sought (Table 4.3). This can be done by feeling the breasts with a soapy hand while washing. The breast awareness approach should allow prompt reassurance to be given in most cases, and increase the likelihood that conservative surgery would be possible if breast cancer were detected. However, it should be remembered that breast awareness has no proven value.

TABLE 4.3

'Breast awareness' – changes for which medical advice should be sought

- Dimpling or flaking of the skin
- Nipple discharge
- New lump or thickening in the breast tissue, particularly if not cyclic
- Unusual pain or discomfort
- Any new difference in the appearance of the breasts (when looking at them, lifting them, or moving the arms)

Key points – diagnosis

- A logical process for assessing breast pain or masses will greatly enhance diagnostic accuracy.
- Clinical examination plus imaging plus cytological or histopathological examination (triple assessment) represent the diagnostic gold standard.
- No test is pathognomonic. Clinical judgment has high value.
- Breast screening programs have modest utility. Their greatest value may be in increasing patient self-awareness and in the improved organization of clinical services.
- Breast self-examination can no longer be recommended, though women should be aware of normal physiological changes and thus be alerted to the first chance observation of a pathological change.

Key references

Baxter N; Canadian Task Force on Preventive Health Care. Preventive health care, 2001 update: should women be routinely taught breast self-examination to screen for breast cancer? *CMAJ* 2001;164:1837–46.

Douek M, Vaidya JS, Lakhani SR et al. Can magnetic-resonance imaging help elucidate natural history of breast cancer multicentricity? *Lancet* 1998;351:801–2.

Jørgensen KJ, Gøtzsche PC. Overdiagnosis in publicly organised mammography screening programmes: systematic review of incidence trends. *BMJ* 2009;339:b2587.

Mettlin CJ, Smart CR. The Canadian National Breast Screening Study. An appraisal and implications for early detection policy. *Cancer* 1993;72:1461–5.

Nekhlyudov L, Fletcher SW. Is it time to stop teaching breast self-examination? *CMAJ* 2001;164:1851.

Nystrom L, Andersson I, Bjurstam N et al. Long-term effects of mammography screening: updated overview of the Swedish randomized trials. *Lancet* 2002;359:909–19.

Tabar L, Fagerberg G, Duffy SW, Day NE. The Swedish two county trial of mammographic screening for breast cancer: recent results and calculation of benefit. *J Epidemiol Community Health* 1989;43:107–14.

Vaidya JS, Vyas JJ, Chinoy RF et al. Multicentricity of breast cancer: whole-organ analysis and clinical implications. *Br J Cancer* 1996;74:820–4.

Walloch J. Technique and interpretation of breast aspiration cytology. *Clin Obstet Gynecol* 1989;32:786–99.

5 Local control of primary tumor

The dogma of the second half of the 20th century, which maintained that local control of breast cancer has no effect on long-term survival, has been overturned as the results of randomized trials have matured. It appears that local control does, indeed, have a significant impact on overall survival, though the mechanism may not be straightforward.

In general, it is currently accepted that the disease originates in the breast, but has more widespread manifestations. The malignant potential of an individual cancer manifests early, and most breast cancers that have the potential to metastasize do so before clinical diagnosis is possible. Long-term follow-up studies have clearly shown that the risks of recurrence and death correlate with disease stage at diagnosis. Thus, the goal of staging is to gather adequate prognostic information to guide therapy, taking into account the associated risks. It is important to establish:
- the origin and type of the tumor including receptor status (estrogen receptor [ER] and human epidermal growth factor receptor [HER-2] are now standard)
- how far the tumor has spread
- other factors, such as menopausal status and the presence of concomitant disease that may influence the treatment plan.

The goals of treatment can be to:
- achieve cure for the individual patient
- prevent or delay recurrence for as long as possible
- relieve symptoms and improve quality of life in patients in whom distant metastases are present at diagnosis (this group accounts for about 10% of new diagnoses in most Western countries).

Therapies such as radiotherapy and surgery are used to achieve local control and prevent distant spread, while other treatments (chemotherapy, immunotherapy, hormonal treatment) are used to alter the systemic milieu and attack distant metastases. Meta-analysis has clearly shown that local treatment does indeed impact on distant control. For every four recurrences prevented locally at 5 years, one life is saved at 15 years; there is a suggestion that this ratio of 4:1 could even increase to 1:1 for low-risk cancers. Local and systemic therapies are not necessarily used sequentially, but are mixed to maximize benefit and minimize risk according to the needs of the individual patient.

Rationale for local treatment

Local treatment for breast cancer consists of surgery and radiotherapy, which aim to remove the cancer, stop its spread and reduce the likelihood of local recurrence within the breast, chest wall or axillary nodes. Systemic therapies, including chemotherapy and hormonal manipulation, reduce the risk of both local and systemic recurrence and, to some extent, improve survival.

Primary breast surgery has long been the first treatment step. Although it has been suggested that primary surgery may be unnecessary, the benefit of removing the primary tumor has been difficult to test in a randomized fashion for obvious ethical reasons. However, two sets of data appear to show that it may be important. First, in randomized trials in elderly women (mostly > 70 years, which may no longer be considered 'elderly'), it was found that primary surgery had a superior outcome compared with primary endocrine therapy with tamoxifen. However, choosing a more suitable subset of these patients with a shorter expectancy of life and using a better endocrine agent, such as an aromatase inhibitor, may achieve an equivalent result. Two trials – Endocrine +/– Surgical Therapy for Elderly women with Mammary cancer (ESTEeM) and Primary Aromatase INhibitor (and other aLternatives) as Effective aS Surgery (PAINLESS) – have been attempting to answer this question, but participation has been poor, mainly because it appears that patients and their doctors usually favor one side or the other in an individual case, losing the equipoise necessary for randomization. The second set of data comes from trials of neoadjuvant chemotherapy in which women received chemotherapy either before or after surgery. The expectation in these trials was that the neoadjuvant chemotherapy, which was initiated at the earliest opportunity, would improve survival. Unfortunately, it did not. Furthermore, neoadjuvant chemotherapy was associated with poorer local control, especially when the surgery was inadequate or when it was omitted altogether because there appeared to be a complete response to the treatment.

A large, albeit retrospective, series reported improved survival in women with bony metastasis following excision of the primary tumor. These data suggest that removal of the tumor or even the tumor-bearing area is important; this may be because it harbors stem cells that are otherwise resistant to either systemic therapy or radiotherapy. Finally, the fact that screening mammography has an effect, albeit very modest, on mortality is good evidence that earlier surgery is superior to later surgery.

Where local control is unlikely to be achieved, as for example in inflammatory carcinomas and extensive local disease, primary surgery may be contraindicated; distant metastases are another relative contraindication. The main indication for primary surgery is the realistic opportunity to achieve long-term disease-free survival or effective cure.

Surgical treatment of primary cancer

The aims of surgical treatment for primary breast cancer are to:
- achieve cure in patients in whom the disease is confined to the breast
- achieve local control of the disease in order to prevent complications, such as skin ulceration
- try to stop any (further) metastatic spread from the primary tumor
- determine the pathological stage of lymph-node involvement
- obtain sufficient tumor for measurement of ER status and other prognostic markers.

Surgery may consist of either mastectomy or conservative procedures, so-called 'lumpectomy' in the USA and wide local excision in the UK (Table 5.1).

Mastectomy. The most commonly used mastectomy procedures are total mastectomy and axillary clearance. In many cases, axillary clearance can be avoided if the sentinel node is found to be negative.

Simple mastectomy. The entire breast tissue, including the axillary tail, is removed together with the skin, nipple and areola (Figure 5.1). Samples from the lowest axillary lymph nodes are usually also taken.

TABLE 5.1
Surgical options in breast cancer

Advantages	Disadvantages

Breast-conserving surgery including sentinel node biopsy only *or* axillary clearance if proven node-positive

• Breast preserved • No significant difference in overall survival • No need for prosthesis	• Postoperative radiotherapy indicated; may be replaced in the future by targeted intraoperative radiotherapy depending on the results of clinical trials • Slightly higher risk of local recurrence than mastectomy • Cosmetic results sometimes disappointing

Total mastectomy with sentinel node biopsy only *or* with axillary clearance if proven node-positive (modified radical mastectomy)

• Postoperative radiotherapy not usually required • Slightly better local control than with breast-conserving surgery	• External prosthesis or reconstruction usually required; reconstruction can be a major operation, albeit with excellent results • Radiotherapy recommended for those with positive nodes (especially > 3). Clinical trials (e.g. SUPREMO) are ongoing for patients at intermediate risk

Classic (Halsted) radical mastectomy (rarely done)

• May help to achieve local control of indolent advanced disease that has failed to respond to radiotherapy or systemic therapy	• Ugly appearance that is difficult to mask with a prosthesis and breast reconstruction is difficult

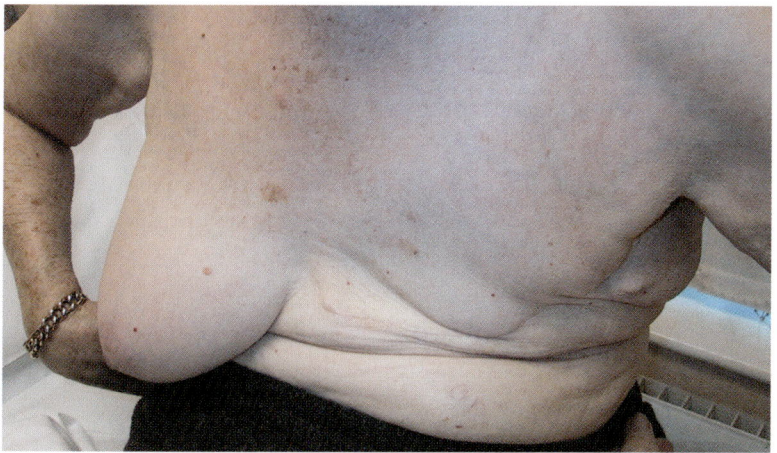

Figure 5.1 The typical appearance following mastectomy in an elderly woman.

Modified radical mastectomy. The classic form of modified radical mastectomy described by Patey removes the same structures as simple mastectomy, together with the pectoralis minor muscle. This allows easy removal of the axillary lymph nodes without greatly increasing the amount of tissue removed. However, most surgeons do not remove the pectoralis minor muscle and retract it to expose the level 3 nodes; the authors' preferred approach is to access the axillary vein from between the major and minor muscles.

Subcutaneous mastectomy. In a small number of women, it is possible to remove most of the breast tissue while leaving the skin and nipple intact. The breast can then be reconstructed immediately with an implant. This procedure is, however, mainly used in women with high-risk precancerous conditions, such as carcinoma in situ. Intraoperative radiotherapy is being tested in an attempt to treat the retained nipple and early results are encouraging.

Skin-sparing mastectomy. When an immediate or delayed reconstruction is planned, the mastectomy can be performed through a smaller circular incision about 1 cm outside the areola; surprisingly, this provides sufficient access to carry out a full axillary clearance with the right instruments and assistance. The skin envelop can be immediately filled with the newly harvested tissue, or with a prosthesis that can be later replaced at a more definitive operation. This approach is not yet considered standard of care; concerns remain about surgical oncological safety, tolerance of radiotherapy and interference with chemotherapy.

Complications. Mastectomy is safe and most patients recover well. The most common complication after surgery is wound infection. However, postoperative bleeding and hematoma are becoming more common as the number of women taking medications for cardiac co-morbidities that alter the normal hemostatic mechanisms increases (clopidogrel being the worst culprit); the risks of stopping such medication need to be balanced against the risk of postoperative bleeding that can occur despite meticulous surgical technique. In general, hematoma can be almost completely avoided by careful attention to surgical hemostasis, with no need to stop aspirin before breast surgery. Arm numbness, shoulder weakness and lymphedema resulting from damage to the lymph nodes is becoming rarer as radical procedures are performed less often. Numbness can be significantly reduced by using a surgical technique to preserve most of the branches of the intercostobrachial nerve, which may help to maintain shoulder movement in conjunction with postoperative physiotherapy (see Chapter 7). Common complications are listed in Table 5.2.

TABLE 5.2

Complications after mastectomy for primary breast cancer

- Wound complications
    - bruising
    - hematoma
    - swelling
    - delayed healing
    - infection
    - damaged intercostal brachial nerve
- Shoulder weakness or stiffness
- Swelling of arm due to lymphedema

Local control of primary tumor

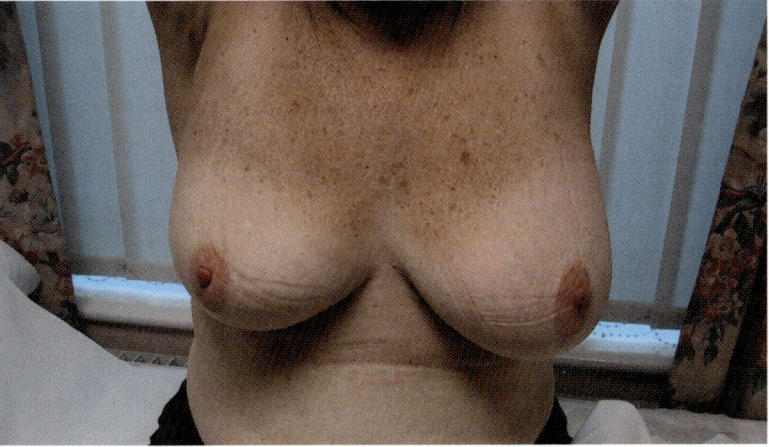

Figure 5.2 The typical appearance after breast-conserving surgery.

Conservative procedures include:
- wide local excision, in which the lump is removed with a 1-cm margin of normal tissue
- quadrantectomy, in which an entire quadrant is removed (Figure 5.2).

With adjuvant radiotherapy, survival following these procedures is comparable with that achieved with mastectomy. The latest overview has shown that breast conservation including radiotherapy has a slightly higher risk of local recurrence than mastectomy, but does not jeopardize overall survival. It should also be recognized that conservative surgery is not suitable for all patients; the outcome is influenced by a number of factors, including the size of the tumor relative to the size of the breast, the stage and grade of the tumor (Table 5.3), and perhaps age.

TABLE 5.3

Breast cancers suitable for conservative surgery

- Single clinical and mammographic lesion
- Tumor ≤ 4 cm
- No local advancement (T1, T2 < 4 cm), extensive nodal involvement (N0, N1), or metastases (M0)
- Tumor > 4 cm in a large breast

Moreover, many women opt for mastectomy because of a need to feel that the tumor has been completely eradicated, or because of an unwillingness to accept adjuvant radiotherapy. In such situations, and especially in women over the age of 45, targeted intraoperative radiotherapy (TARGIT) offers the possibility of avoiding a mastectomy. TARGIT is currently being evaluated in an international randomized trial involving over 2000 patients (www.targit.org.uk) with accrual completed in March 2010.

Choice of operation. This should be discussed fully with the patient, and a considered decision should be made. Ideally, there should be more than one consultation with the surgeon and the radiation oncologist should attend if possible.

It is the patient's short-term and long-term satisfaction with the overall treatment as well as the objective cancer control outcome, rather than the proportion of breast cancers undergoing conservation, that should be a measure of quality of care.

Treatment of regional lymph nodes

The indications for axillary surgery and the extent to which it should be carried out in women with operable breast cancer remain controversial; the dogma of axillary clearance is now being replaced by a dogma for sentinel node biopsy. Clinicians who have observed uncontrolled axillary disease are cautious of taking any steps that could risk such an outcome. In terms of local control, however, there may be little to choose between the success of surgery and the success of radiotherapy, balanced against the relatively rare, but significant, morbidity of either approach. It is likely that axillary clearance will have a decreasing role in the future, partly because of the earlier presentation of breast cancer and partly because of improvements in the prognostic value of tumor markers.

Axillary clearance. If axillary dissection is necessary, the technique used must aim to minimize the morbidity of the procedure as much as possible. One of the most distressing postoperative problems is anesthesia or paresthesia in the axilla and the medial aspect of the arm, which results from surgical division of the intercostobrachial nerve. In skilled hands, this complication is easily avoided. Restriction of shoulder movement is less of a problem if the pectoralis minor is not divided.

A standard axillary clearance should involve excision of only those tissues anterior and inferior to the axillary vein, leaving behind the lymphatics that drain the arm, which are usually thought to be situated above the vein. A novel approach to identifying the arm lymphatics using a blue dye injected in the forearm/hand has shown that some of the vessels draining the arm are in fact below the axillary vein and could be saved during axillary clearance by intraoperative identification.

As about 26% of lymph nodes are expected to be positive, the number needed to treat (NNT) to prevent 1 additional bad outcome is about 4 (100/26). This is much lower than the NNT for most other treatments used in medicine, and is an order of magnitude lower than the NNTs for other treatments used for breast cancer. Thus, the sentinel node biopsy (see below) is especially important when the background risk of node positivity is low (e.g. 10%). In such cases, the NNT with axillary clearance would be high (NNT = 100/10 = 10) and the effect of false-negative sentinel node biopsy would be clinically insignificant.

With increasing use of sentinel node biopsy, lymphedema of the arm is now relatively uncommon. Radiotherapy should not be given after a full axillary clearance; although it is often used in the presence extranodal spread, its value is not well established.

Prognosis. The role of the axillary dissection to establish the prognosis and thereby to help select appropriate systemic therapy has been contentious mainly because of the unnecessary morbidity associated with a negative axillary clearance. However, the increasing use of sentinel node biopsy has made axillary clearance a significantly safer procedure. The current recommendation is to perform a complete axillary clearance if a sentinel node is involved.

Sentinel node biopsy is the 'standard of care' in many parts of the world. It is now recognized that most breast cancers spread in a predictable path along the axillary lymphatics with the lowermost node in the chain (the sentinel node) being the first to be affected. In the procedure, radiolabeled colloid or a patent blue dye is injected subdermally under the areola. A path can then be traced to the first draining lymph node in the axilla (the definition of a sentinel node), which is independent of the location of the tumor in the breast. Intraoperative assessment of the lymph node is possible with imprint cytology. If the sentinel node is negative, it is reasonable not to explore the axilla further. If positive, formal axillary dissection is justified. The biological basis of this procedure is that examining the axillary nodes provides prognostic information about the risk of systemic recurrence. A negative sentinel node with skip lesions higher up the axilla occurs in only about 3% of cases in the hands of a skilled surgeon. This low false-negative rate is achieved by meticulous technique and by not ignoring suspicious enlarged nodes found near the sentinel node intraoperatively.

Two new techniques hold promise of being as sensitive as imprint cytology (70–80%), but without the need for an experienced pathologist. One is to use reverse transcription polymerase chain reaction and assess the amplification of CK17 and mammoglobin that are only found if breast cancer cells are present in the lymph node. The other is to use the differential scattering of visible light by the tumor tissue and normal lymph-node tissue.

It is possible, if not probable, that equal or better prognostic information will be gained from the primary tumor as well as molecular examination of the sentinel node in the future.

Studies have reported a significant reduction in morbidity, and an improvement in quality of life and patient satisfaction, after sentinel node biopsy. However, long-term local recurrence results are yet to be reported.

Expertise and experience in the sentinel node procedure are implicit requirements. Major institutions have tended to require surgeons to have performed sentinel node biopsy followed by axillary dissection in a substantial number of patients in order to achieve an acceptable standard of expertise, unless it was part of their surgical training. It should be remembered that the technique has been tested mainly in patients with clinically negative axilla. Also, the follow-up of sentinel node biopsy trials is still short, and only long-term follow-up will show the exact additional risks of local and distant failures because of possible undertreatment of axilla. The temptation to use the technique in every case should be avoided.

When discussing axillary surgery with the patient, the following issues need to be discussed:
- the effect of false-negative sentinel node biopsy in relation to the background node-positivity risk
- the risk of a second operation if the sentinel node is positive and if intraoperative assessment of the lymph node is either unavailable or falsely negative (20–30% in most cases)
- the morbidity of axillary clearance in general and in the hands of the surgeon.

Reconstructive surgery

Breast reconstruction following mastectomy is becoming increasingly popular, though currently only about 5% of patients undergo such surgery. The aims of reconstructive surgery are to:
- restore the natural breast contour as far as possible
- establish symmetry between the new mound and the remaining breast
- to produce a pleasing nipple–areola complex.

Ideally, breast reconstruction should be performed at the same time as the initial mastectomy as this reduces the psychological impact of losing a breast and avoids the need for further surgery. In practice, however, this may not be feasible, as both a cancer surgeon and a plastic surgeon are needed. A number of options for breast reconstruction are available (Table 5.4).

TABLE 5.4
Options for breast reconstruction

- Silicone gel implants
- Tissue expanders and prostheses
- Myocutaneous flaps
    - latissimus dorsi
    - transverse rectus abdominis

Silicone gel implants offer the simplest approach to reconstruction, and are suitable for women with small breasts. The implant is placed high on the chest wall, beneath the pectoralis major muscle. The full effect is not achieved until several months after surgery, when the skin and surrounding tissues have stretched to accommodate the implant. Careful adjustment of the size and position of the remaining breast is necessary to achieve a symmetrical appearance. There is no scientific evidence that silicone implants are associated with any health hazard, including autoimmune disease.

Tissue expanders. This approach involves implanting an inflatable bag which is filled with saline via a subcutaneous valve implanted in the patient's side. About 50 mL of saline is injected at 1–2-week intervals, until the breast mound is about 1.5 times larger than the remaining breast (so that the breast will hang naturally when the bag is removed). The bag is then removed and replaced with a silicone implant at a second operation. Recent devices such as the Becker prosthesis incorporate a silicone prosthesis (Figure 5.3) and so only the valve needs to be removed, which can be done under local anesthetic.

Myocutaneous flaps. This technique involves using a flap of skin and muscle to recreate the breast mound. This approach is useful in women with large breasts, those in whom a large amount of tissue was removed, or in cases where the skin is unlikely to accommodate an implant (e.g.

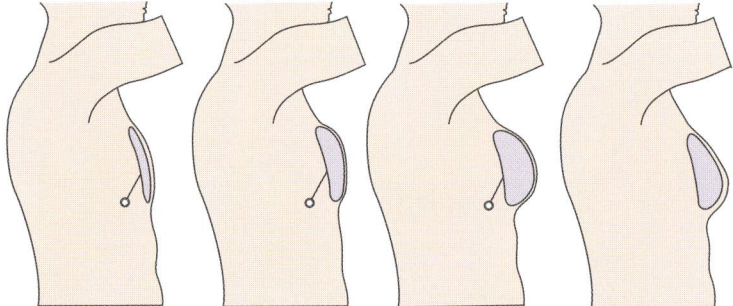

Figure 5.3 In the Becker breast reconstruction technique, a silicone prosthesis containing a tissue expander filled via a subcutaneous valve is used to create a new breast mound. The valve is subsequently removed under local anesthetic.

Local control of primary tumor

after radiotherapy). The two most common reconstructions involve the rectus abdominis (transverse rectus abdominis myocutaneous [TRAM] flap) or latissimus dorsi muscles (Figure 5.4).

Deep inferior epigastric artery perforator (DIEP) flap. Immediate breast reconstruction after mastectomy is most commonly achieved

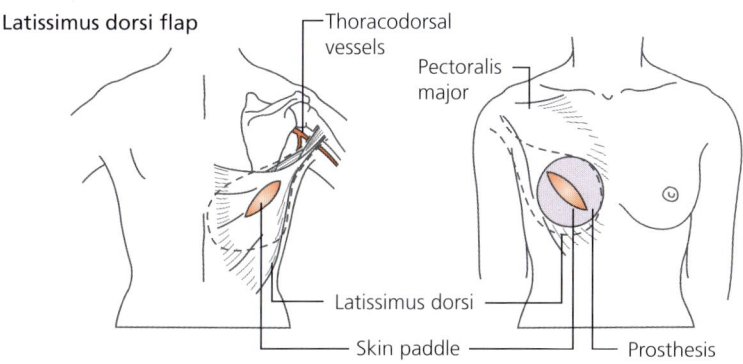

Figure 5.4 Breast reconstruction by myocutaneous flap can involve either a latissimus dorsi or transverse rectus abdominis myocutaneous (TRAM) flap.

using adipose tissue from the abdomen harvested with its blood supply (the DIEP flap). This technique spares most of the rectus abdominis muscle and uses delicate arterial anastomosis without jeopardizing the donor site. The procedure can take several hours and can achieve a nearly symmetrical breast. Research into sensory innervation of such a breast is ongoing. It is important, however, to appreciate that the operation usually lasts 6–8 hours and further, smaller operations are also often required to correct minor defects.

Nipple reconstruction. If desired, the nipple can be reconstructed surgically to give a reasonable cosmetic appearance. Tissue can be taken from the other nipple or, if necessary, from the thigh or labia. This operation should be performed several months after mastectomy to allow the reconstructed breast to attain its final shape, so that the heights of the nipples can be matched.

Radiotherapy

Radiotherapy is considered mandatory for most patients undergoing conservative surgery, and is considered appropriate for women at high risk of recurrence after mastectomy, such as:

- women with a large primary tumor, particularly if the tumor is poorly differentiated
- women with lymph-node involvement who have not undergone full axillary clearance
- women with involvement of the pectoralis major muscle.

Treatment is normally given in 3–5-weekly sessions for up to 6 weeks. The most common side effects are skin reactions and, occasionally, nausea and vomiting; pneumonitis resulting from irradiation of the lung occurs in fewer than 2% of patients. Older regimens inadvertently included the heart and the anterior descending coronary artery, and caused an excess cardiac mortality which was most conspicuous in those with left-sided breast cancers. Newer regimens, including intensity-modulated radiotherapy, are expected to reduce the cardiac dose and consequently the morbidity.

Meta-analysis data released in late 2004, covering 79 trials (about 42 000 women over a period as long as 20 years), have yielded the following conclusions.

- Radiotherapy provides highly effective local control, preventing local recurrence in more than 80% of those treated.
- Cardiac side effects can be significant, but the trend is to fewer complications with modern treatment approaches.

It is worth noting again, here, that for every four recurrences prevented at 5 years, one life is saved at 15 years. However, a new analysis suggests that this ratio of 4:1 varies with the stage of the primary tumor and that, for smaller cancers with a good prognosis, the ratio is 1:1 (i.e. for every local recurrence prevented, one life is saved; see page 28). Thus, there is even more reason to ensure that small breast cancers receive the best local treatment, because any local recurrence appears to be detrimental to overall survival.

Hypofractionated radiotherapy. A large trial in Canada and the Standardisation of Radiotherapy (START) trials in the UK have shown that the breast is more sensitive to fraction size than previously thought. The START Trial B found that a 3-week regimen gave equivalent results to a conventional 6-week regimen in local recurrence rates at 5-year follow-up. This has prompted the 'faster radiotherapy for breast cancer patients' trial that is testing whether 1 week of therapy can be as good and without side effects. Of course, the ultimate hypofractionation is to give the radiotherapy in a single dose intraoperatively and targeted to tumor bed.

Targeted intraoperative radiotherapy is used following local excision of early breast cancer. It has been developed over the last 10 years and is being tested in randomized trials. The Intrabeam system, which was developed at University College, London, UK, is a completely portable unit that can be used in a standard operating theater to deliver targeted radiotherapy (Figure 5.5; www.targit.org.uk).

TARGIT is of great potential value in the management of early breast cancer treated by breast-conserving techniques. Modern understanding of breast cancer pathology now suggests that occult/latent lesions in areas of the breast remote from the index quadrant are not the reason for local relapse, which almost always occurs at the site of the original excision. (Indeed, as has already been pointed out, a cancer is just as likely to develop in the contralateral breast as a recurrence outside the index quadrant in the ipsilateral breast, yet we would never consider prophylactic radiotherapy to the other side!) If that is indeed the case,

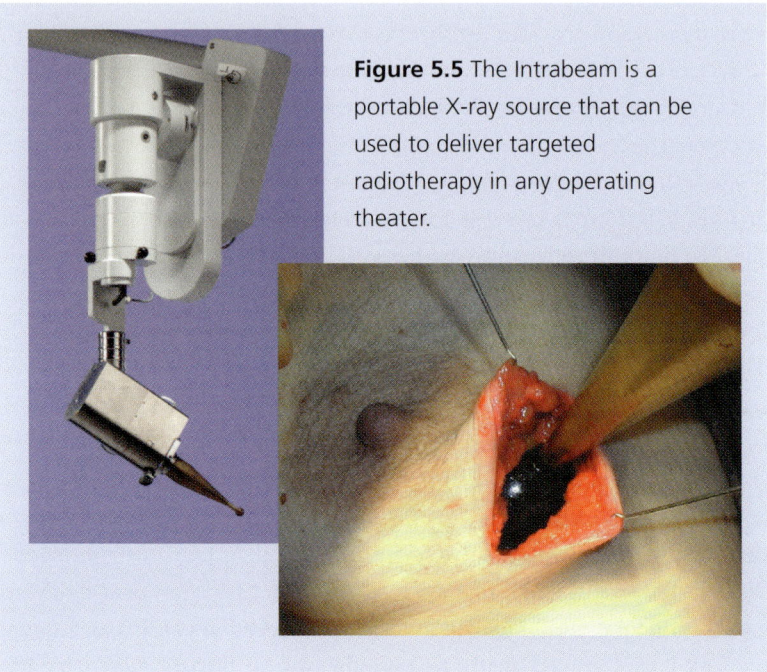

Figure 5.5 The Intrabeam is a portable X-ray source that can be used to deliver targeted radiotherapy in any operating theater.

then carefully targeted high-dose radiotherapy at the time of surgery may obviate the need for external-beam therapy, thus saving machine time and the patient's time. In addition, it opens up the possibility of breast conservation for breast cancer among women in the developing world; in most developing countries and many parts of the developed world, journeys are so long and/or tiring as to make breast-conserving surgery a non-viable option. Furthermore, by applying the walls of the excision cavity to the applicator after tumorectomy, the conformal geometry is much better than the simulations required for external-beam treatment, which should in theory lead to better local control of the disease.

Translational research has shown that postoperative wound fluid normally stimulates cancer cell growth, motility and invasiveness (commensurate with the need to heal the wound). TARGIT has been found to abrogate this effect of surgical wounding. Thus, in addition to reaching the right tissues, TARGIT is also applied at the right time. This biological rationale is perhaps borne out in the clinic. The first series that used TARGIT was started in 1998 and accrued 300 patients. These patients received TARGIT, as well as external-beam radiotherapy. The actuarial local recurrence rates in this unselected group of patients have been very low – 1.5% at 5 years. From the case mix, the estimated local recurrence in this group of patients would be expected to be at least 4–5%. The ongoing TARGIT-B trial will determine if TARGIT boost is superior to conventional externally delivered boost dose to the tumor bed.

Early results from the TARGIT-A trial, which is nearing its accrual goal (n = 2232), are expected in June 2010. If TARGIT becomes the standard of care, as its single dose would substitute for the usual 3–6 weeks' postoperative course of radiotherapy, it will save many women from losing their breasts and reduce healthcare costs. And in high-risk, especially young, women, a tumor bed boost with TARGIT has the potential to reduce local recurrence rates.

Other techniques with a similar rationale include 'ELIOT' (ELectron IntraOperative Therapy), which was developed in the European breast cancer center in Milan, and the Mobitron system.

The MammoSite technique uses a balloon catheter inserted in the site to deliver brachytherapy. The Xoft is a hybrid between Intrabeam and MammoSite, but clinical experience in its use is very limited.

All these techniques offer different advantages and in addition to the outcome of randomized controlled trials, individual centers may offer one or more to best fit the patient's needs.

Key points – local control of primary tumor

- Mastectomy and lumpectomy plus radiation are therapeutically equivalent for most women.
- Given adequate information, women can choose equally between mastectomy and breast conservation approaches.
- Breast reconstruction is viable and can be offered as an immediate or a delayed procedure.
- In the future, selected patients may be able to avoid 6 weeks of conventional postoperative radiotherapy by receiving a single dose of partial breast radiotherapy in the intra- or perioperative period.

Key references

Association of Breast Surgery at BASO 2009. Surgical guidelines for the management of breast cancer. *EJSO* 2009;35:S1–22.

Breast Surgeons Group of the British Association of Surgical Oncology. Guidelines for surgeons in the management of symptomatic breast disease in the United Kingdom. *Eur J Surg Oncol* 1995;21:1–13.

Coombs N, Chen W, Taylor R, Boyages J. A decision tool for predicting sentinel node accuracy from breast tumor size and grade. *Breast J* 2007;13:593–8.

Early Breast Cancer Trialists' Collaborative Group. Effects of radiotherapy and of differences in the extent of surgery for early breast cancer on local recurrence and 15-year survival: an overview of the randomised trials. *Lancet* 2005;366:2087–2106.

Goldhirsch A, Wood WC, Senn H-J et al. Meeting highlights: International Consensus Panel on the Treatment of Primary Breast Cancer. *J Natl Cancer Inst* 1995;87:1441–5.

Houghton J, Baum M, Haybittle JL. Role of radiotherapy following total mastectomy in patients with early breast cancer. The Closed Trials Working Party of the CRC Breast Cancer Trials Group. *World J Surg* 1994;18:117–22.

Kyndi M, Sørensen FB, Knudsen H et al. Estrogen receptor, progesterone receptor, HER-2, and response to postmastectomy radiotherapy in high-risk breast cancer: the Danish Breast Cancer Cooperative Group. *J Clin Oncol* 2008:26;1419–26.

Sacks NP, Baum M. Primary management of carcinoma of the breast. *Lancet* 1993;342:1402–8.

Sainsbury R, Haward B, Rider L et al. Influence of clinician workload and patterns of treatment on survival from breast cancer. *Lancet* 1995;345: 1265–70.

Vaidya JS, Dewar JA, Brown DC, Thompson AM. A mathematical model for the effect of a false-negative sentinel node biopsy on breast cancer mortality: a tool for everyday use. *Breast Cancer Res* 2005;7:225–7.

Vaidya JS, Tobias JS, Baum M et al. Targeted intraoperative radiotherapy (TARGIT) yields very low recurrence rates when given as a boost. *Int J Rad Oncol Biol Phys* 2006;66: 1335–8.

Vaidya JS, Tobias JS, Baum M et al. Intraoperative radiotherapy for breast cancer. *Lancet Oncol* 2004;5:165–73.

Veronesi U, Paganelli G, Galimberti V et al. Sentinel-node biopsy to avoid axillary node dissection in breast cancer with clinically negative lymph nodes. *Lancet* 1997;349:1864–7.

6 Adjuvant therapy

While surgery and radiotherapy offer control of the primary tumor, systemic estrogen therapies aim to prevent or delay distant metastases. This is called adjuvant therapy and marks the most significant change in breast cancer management in the past 25 years. Data have shown unequivocally that adjuvant therapy provides a significant and prolonged improvement in survival. Indeed, the approximately 30% fall in breast cancer mortality in the UK and USA since 1985 (from an all-time high in the late 1970s) has mainly been ascribed to the widespread adoption of adjuvant systemic therapy.

Adjuvant therapy is based on the principle that breast cancer is, for many women, a systemic disease at the time of diagnosis with undetectable dormant micrometastases. These micrometastases may develop into clinically relevant metastases years after primary diagnosis. Some studies have demonstrated the presence of circulating tumor cells in the blood or bone marrow at the time of diagnosis of the primary breast cancer, using sensitive techniques such as polymerase chain reaction, but the significance of these cells is uncertain and some are not clonogenic. There is considerable interest in using circulating tumor cells to monitor the effectiveness of adjuvant treatment and also to predict those patients who might relapse; however, this remains a research tool rather than standard practice. Characteristics of the primary tumor that may predict the risk of metastatic disease in individual women include the involvement of lymph nodes in the axilla (and the number of lymph nodes), high histological grade of the primary tumor and large tumor size. The hazard rates for relapse (time of and likelihood of) vary according to these and other factors. The aim of adjuvant treatment is to eliminate micrometastatic disease, thereby reducing the risk of relapse and death.

The first systemic approaches to preventing recurrence were hormonal. The general principle was to deprive the tumor of estrogen, thereby altering the hormonal milieu. This was followed by the use of cytotoxic drugs as adjuvant treatment based on the success of treating leukemia and lymphoma in the 1960s and metastatic breast cancer in the 1970s.

With the identification of the estrogen receptors and progesterone receptors on breast cancer cells in the 1970s, it became possible to stratify tumors into those most likely to respond to hormone therapy and those unlikely to do so. As it happened, most hormone-receptor-positive cancers were found in postmenopausal women and hormone-receptor-negative disease was more likely in younger women. This led to the generalization that chemotherapy would be most widely applicable in premenopausal women and hormonal therapy in postmenopausal women. Subsequent research has refined this approach and age, per se, is not the main determinant of therapy. Indeed, many women with hormone-receptor-positive disease will receive both chemotherapy and hormonal therapy, whereas women with hormone-receptor-negative disease are candidates for only chemotherapy. Moreover, the *level* of expression of the estrogen receptor (ER) and/or progesterone receptor can be used to identify endocrine-responsive patients, further refining the choice of therapy together with other factors, such as expression of human epidermal growth factor receptor 2 (HER2) (Tables 6.1 and 6.2). Subsequent research has identified the importance of growth factors such as HER2, which is a target for therapy with the monoclonal antibody trastuzumab.

Hormonal therapy

Tamoxifen was developed as a fertility drug in the 1970s and has subsequently become the mainstay of treatment for breast cancer. Treatment with tamoxifen for 5 years reduces the relative risk of dying from breast cancer in both pre- and postmenopausal women. Tamoxifen works as a selective estrogen receptor modulator, and has effects both as an estrogen agonist and antagonist depending on the tissue and receptor type. In breast tissue, tamoxifen blocks the peripheral actions of estrogen (Figure 6.1). Tamoxifen binds competitively with 17-β-estradiol at the receptor site, producing a nuclear complex that decreases DNA synthesis and inhibits estrogen, causing cells to remain in the G0 and G1 phases of the cell cycle. Tamoxifen is a prodrug, which is metabolized in the liver by the cytochrome P450 isoform CYP2 D6 and CYP3a4 into

TABLE 6.1

St Gallen recommendations 2009: thresholds for treatment modalities

Treatment modality	Indication	Comments
Endocrine therapy	Any ER staining	ER negative and PgR positive are probably artefactual
Anti-HER2 therapy	HER2 positive (>30% intense and complete staining [IHC] or FISH >2.2+)*	May use clinical trial definitions
Chemotherapy		
In HER2-positive disease (with anti-HER2 therapy)	Trial evidence for trastuzumab is limited to use with or following chemotherapy*	Combined endocrine therapy + anti-HER2 therapy without chemotherapy in strongly ER-positive HER2-positive is logical but unproven
In triple-negative disease	Most patients*†	No proven alternative; most at elevated risk
In ER-positive, HER2-negative disease (with endocrine therapy)	Variable according to risk*	

*Patients with tumors <1 cm without axillary nodal involvement and other features indicating increased metastatic potential (e.g. vascular invasion) might not need adjuvant systemic therapy. Endocrine therapy should be considered if the tumor is, however, endocrine responsive.
†Medullary carcinoma, apocrine carcinoma, and adenoid cystic carcinoma do not require chemotherapy due to low risk despite being triple negative (provided there is no axillary node involvement and no other signs of increased metastatic risk).
ER, estrogen receptor; IHC, immunohistochemistry; PgR, progesterone receptor.
Reproduced by permission of Oxford University Press from Goldhirsch A, Ingle JN, Gelber RD et al; Panel members. Thresholds for therapies: highlights of the St Gallen International Expert Consensus on the primary therapy of early breast cancer 2009. *Ann Oncol* 2009;20:1319–29.

active metabolites, such as 4-hydroxytamoxifen and endoxifen, which have 30–100 times greater affinity for the ER than tamoxifen itself.

TABLE 6.2

St Gallen recommendations 2009: chemoendocrine therapy in patients with ER-positive HER2-negative disease

Clinicopathological features	Relative indications for chemoendocrine therapy	Factors not useful for decision	Relative indications for endocrine therapy alone
ER and PgR	Lower ER and PgR level		Higher ER and PgR level
Histological grade	Grade 3	Grade 2	Grade 1
Proliferation*	High	Intermediate	Low
Nodes	Node positive (≥ 4 involved nodes)	Node positive (1–3 involved nodes)	Node negative
PVI	Presence of extensive PVI		Absence of extensive PVI
pT size	> 5 cm	2.1–5 cm	≤ 2 cm
Patient preference	Use all available treatments		Avoid chemotherapy-related side effects
Multigene assays			
Gene signature†	High score	Intermediate score	Low score

*Conventional measures of proliferation include assessment of Ki67-labeling index and pathological description of the frequency of mitoses.
†May assist in deciding whether to add chemotherapy in cases where its use was uncertain after consideration of conventional markers.
ER, estrogen receptor; PgR, progesterone receptor; pT, pathological tumor size; PVI, peritumoral vascular invasion.
Reproduced by permission of Oxford University Press from Goldhirsch A, Ingle JN, Gelber RD et al; Panel members. Thresholds for therapies: highlights of the St Gallen International Expert Consensus on the primary therapy of early breast cancer 2009. *Ann Oncol* 2009;20:1319–29.

Adjuvant therapy

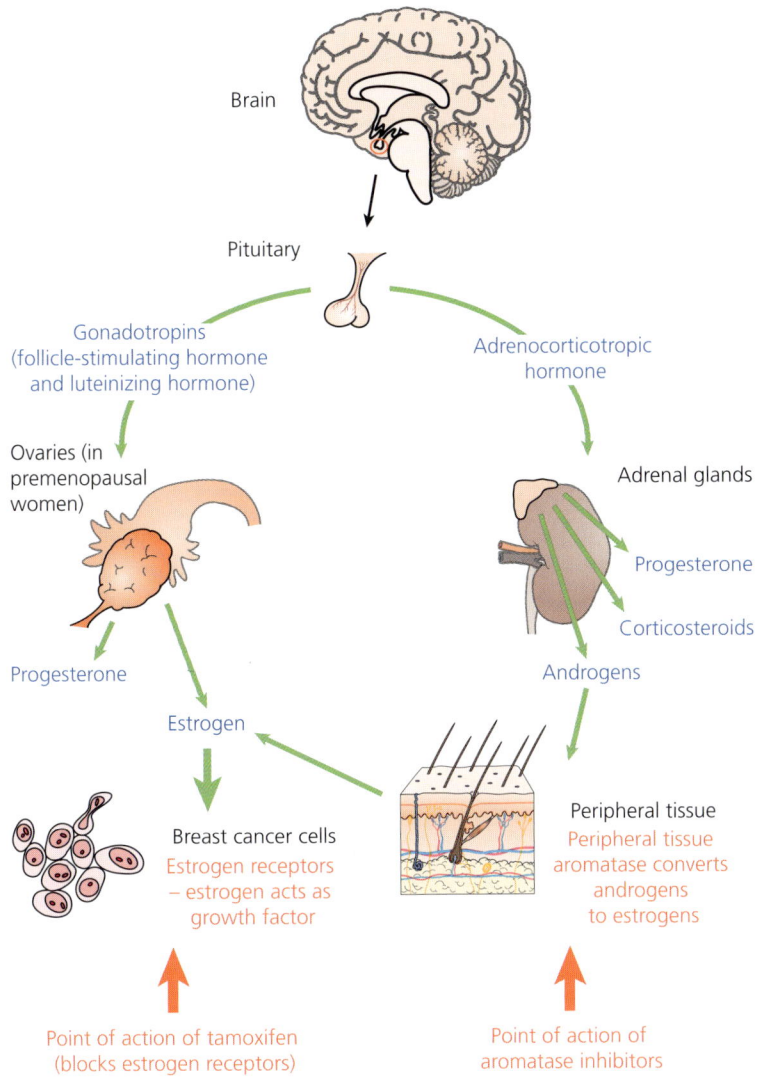

Figure 6.1 Tamoxifen and raloxifene act peripherally by binding to the surface estrogen receptors present in tissue, blocking estrogen itself from binding and initiating a series of steps leading to proliferation. In contrast, the aromatase inhibitors block production of estrogen.

The first trial to show a benefit of adjuvant tamoxifen was the Nolvadex Adjuvant Trial Organisation (NATO) trial, published in 1983, in which 1100 women were randomized after mastectomy to no systemic treatment or tamoxifen 20 mg daily for 2 years. At 66 months of follow-up, the tamoxifen group had a 36% reduction in recurrence and 29% reduction in mortality (Figure 6.2). Subsequent trials confirmed these results in both pre- and postmenopausal women, and showed that tamoxifen reduced the incidence of local recurrence, distant metastases and contralateral breast cancer.

The reduction in the incidence of cancer in the contralateral breast has led to trials investigating tamoxifen as a preventive agent in women considered to be at high risk of developing breast cancer. These trials have been subjected to quinquennial review by the Early Breast Cancer Trialists' Collaborative Group (EBCTCG), which demonstrated in 1990 that women under 50 years of age who were given tamoxifen had a 12% reduction in the risk for disease recurrence and a non-significant reduction in mortality. The figures were even better in postmenopausal women aged over 50 years in whom the reduction in the risk of recurrence was 29% and in the risk of mortality was 20%. Subsequent reviews have confirmed this benefit and tamoxifen has been the standard of care for 5 years.

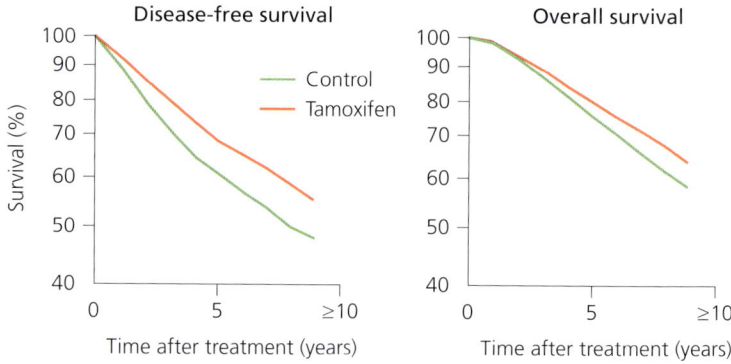

Figure 6.2 Treatment with tamoxifen 20 mg daily significantly improves disease-free and overall survival. The curves continue to separate even after tamoxifen has been stopped.

Two large scale trials – Adjuvant Tamoxifen Treatment Offer More (ATTOM) and Adjuvant Tamoxifen Longer Against Shorter (ATLAS) – have compared the benefits of tamoxifen for 5 vs 10 years. Although the most recent report of the ATTOM trial suggested a trend towards a benefit from continuing tamoxifen, there is not yet sufficient evidence to support the use of tamoxifen beyond 5 years.

Side effects. Tamoxifen has partial estrogen agonist activity, which may cause gynecologic symptoms, such as vaginal bleeding and endometrial polyps, and an increase in endometrial thickness. There is a small but definite 2.5-fold increase in the risk of endometrial cancer; however, this equates to only 1 case in every 1000 women treated for 5 years. The relative risk of thromboembolic disease (deep vein thrombosis and pulmonary emboli) is also slightly increased at 1.6, and is more commonly seen in women over 50 years of age or with a predisposition to venous thrombosis (in which case tamoxifen should be avoided). Recently, patients with a variant form of the *CYP2D6* gene, which is involved in tamoxifen metabolism, have been identified who may not receive full benefit from tamoxifen, because metabolism into its active metabolites (e.g. endoxifen) is too slow. The use of selective serotonin re-uptake inhibitors may decrease the effectiveness of tamoxifen by competing with the CYP2D6 enzyme.

Patients may also experience vasomotor symptoms, such as hot flashes, but there is some evidence that the development of such symptoms may in fact correlate with a better response to treatment due to rapid tamoxifen metabolism.

Resistance. Tamoxifen function can be regulated by a number of variables including growth factors, such as insulin-like growth factor and HER2. In breast tissue, tamoxifen is an ER antagonist and prevents the transcription of ER genes. Patients may become resistant to tamoxifen and relapse during or after completion of therapy. The reasons for resistance are unclear, as tumors usually remain ER-positive. Mechanisms of resistance may include changes in the expression of ER-α or ER-β, alterations in co-regulatory proteins and the effects of cellular kinase signal transduction pathways. Patients with ER-positive breast cancer, which is also HER2-positive, may become resistant to tamoxifen through downregulation of the ER and reduced signaling of kinases lower down the metabolic pathway, including the phosphoinositide-3 and mitogen-activated protein kinase pathways.

Aromatase inhibitors. Circulating levels of estrogen are lower in postmenopausal women than in premenopausal women. However, estrogen is still produced by the aromatization of adrenal androgens by the aromatase enzyme system, which is found mainly in subcutaneous fat but also in muscle, liver and skin. The aromatase enzyme system is therefore a target for inhibition and thus reduction in estrogen biosynthesis in postmenopausal women. Before the menopause, the high levels of estrogen produced by ovarian tissue mean that blocking aromatization in peripheral tissues, such as fat, has little impact on the large amounts estrogen already circulating.

Aromatase inhibitors are divided into two classes.
- Class 1 are steroidal compounds, which are analogs of the natural substrate androstenedione (e.g. exemestane).
- Class 2 are non-steroidal compounds that bind to the heme portion of the cytochrome P450 enzyme, thereby excluding natural substrate from the enzyme (e.g. anastrozole and letrozole).

Both classes of aromatase inhibitor have established superiority over tamoxifen in metastatic breast cancer and have therefore been evaluated as adjuvant therapy. Overall, trials have shown an improvement in disease-free survival (DFS) and some have shown an improvement in survival in postmenopausal women with early breast cancer. Recommendations have therefore been made that this class of drugs should be considered as part of the treatment strategy for all postmenopausal women with breast cancer.

There are three treatment strategies:
- upfront therapy – aromatase inhibitor for 5 years instead of tamoxifen
- switch or planned sequence – aromatase inhibitor started at 2–3 years after tamoxifen
- extended adjuvant therapy – aromatase inhibitor started after 5 years of tamoxifen.

Upfront therapy. The Arimidex, Tamoxifen Alone or in Combination (ATAC) trial was the first to compare a modern aromatase inhibitor, anastrozole, with tamoxifen as initial treatment in postmenopausal women with early breast cancer. A unique feature of this trial was the inclusion of a combination arm, which evaluated both drugs given together. Early follow-up demonstrated superiority for anastrozole over tamoxifen in terms of DFS at 33 months. As expected, no benefit was seen in the hormone-receptor-negative population, which comprised 10% of the study population. Also, no benefit was seen with combination therapy leading to early closure of the study arm; this may have been due to the fact that, in an estrogen-deprived environment produced by anastrozole, tamoxifen is 'seen' as an agonist, restoring estrogen stimulation to breast cancer, whereas in a normal estrogen-rich environment, tamoxifen can exert its classic anti-estrogen effect. The benefit of anastrozole was confirmed at 100 months of follow-up with significant prolongation of DFS, and a significant reduction in distant metastases (424 events vs 487 events; HR 0.86) and contralateral breast cancers (61 events vs 87 events; HR 0.68). (The absolute differences have increased over time and beyond the treatment period indicating a crossover effect. So far, no survival benefit has been demonstrated in this study.) Almost all patients completed the treatment schedule and fewer withdrawals occurred in the anastrozole arm than in the tamoxifen arm, reflecting a more favorable side-effect profile with fewer gynecologic problems and vascular events. There was, however, an increase in the incidence of arthralgia and fractures in the anastrozole arm. The interesting point is that although the beneficial effect persists, the fracture risk was not higher after stopping treatment.

The Breast International Group (BIG) 1-98 trial compared the efficacy and safety of letrozole and tamoxifen, either upfront or in a planned sequence after 2 years. In the primary analysis, there was an 18% (HR 0.82) reduction in the risk of an event at 25.8 months of follow-up in the 8000 women assigned to tamoxifen as initial therapy compared with those assigned to letrozole as initial therapy. This was maintained in the 51-month analysis of women assigned to monotherapy with either tamoxifen or letrozole. There was a significant decrease in distant metastases and contralateral breast cancer. Analysis of the sequential therapies found no difference between the two therapies or between either therapy and monotherapy with letrozole. Early relapses were higher in those assigned to tamoxifen followed by letrozole compared with letrozole monotherapy.

In the ATAC trial, no significant effect on survival has yet been seen. In BIG 1-98, a non-significant decrease was seen in systemic DFS at 51 months in favor of letrozole, but no impact on overall survival has been observed. It is possibly too soon to see a survival difference emerge, especially as patients in both trials had a relatively good prognosis and thus differences in survival would not be expected to emerge at 8–10 years of follow-up. Even at 100 months of follow-up, no survival difference was seen in the ATAC trial, which may well reflect the competing causes of death in this relatively older population that obscure the small survival difference that may have been achieved with anastrozole.

Switch or planned sequence. There is sometimes confusion about these two terms. In a switch trial, patients change from, for example, tamoxifen therapy to an aromatase inhibitor after 2 years (having initially been planned to receive tamoxifen for 5 years) whereas, in a sequence trial, the change is planned at the start with patients receiving tamoxifen for 2–3 years and then changed to an aromatase inhibitor. A number of such trials have been performed.

In the Intergroup Exemestane Study, 4724 women received tamoxifen for an average of 28 months before switching to exemestane. At a median follow-up of 55.7 months, there was a 24% improvement in DFS with exemestane compared with tamoxifen, and an absolute difference at 5 years of 3.3%. In the Austrian Breast and Colorectal Cancer Study Group Trial 8, the Arimidex-Nolvadex Trial 95 and the Italian trials, patients were randomized to receive anastrozole for 3 years after tamoxifen for 2 years. At a median follow-up of 30 months, anastrozole was associated with a decrease in the risk of relapse of 40%. In this study, higher levels of ER or progesterone receptor were predictive of longer relapse-free and overall survival.

Extended adjuvant therapy. The recognition that hormone-receptor-positive breast cancer carries a protracted risk over time, with some patients relapsing 5–15 years after diagnosis (with indeed more deaths after 5 years than before), has led to interest in treatment with endocrine therapy beyond 5 years.

The National Canadian Cancer Institute MA-17 trial was a double-blind placebo-controlled trial in over 5000 postmenopausal women with ER-positive breast cancer, who were disease free after standard treatment with tamoxifen for 5 years. The women were randomized to receive either placebo or letrozole for a further 5 years. The primary endpoint was DFS. This trial was stopped early after the first interim analysis at a median follow-up of 2.4 years, because the results were greatly superior in favor of extended treatment with letrozole than had been expected. At this time point, 1115 patients had been followed-up for more than 40 months and letrozole improved the 4-year DFS by 42% from 89.9% in the placebo arm to 94.4% in the letrozole arm, with a clinically meaningful and significant improvement in long-term DFS. The trial was unblinded and many women crossed over to receive letrozole.

A further trial (National Surgical Adjuvant Breast and Bowel Project 33) was also conducted in postmenopausal women who were disease free after receiving tamoxifen for 5 years and who were then randomized to receive exemestane or placebo. This trial was closed to accrual when the results of the MA-17 trial became available, the treatment arms were unblinded and patients who had been in the placebo arm were offered exemestane. Despite the results of the MA-17 trial, only 560 of 783 women in the exemestane arm continued to receive exemestane and only 344 of 779 women in the placebo arm switched to exemestane. Even with the crossover, exemestane still showed a borderline statistically significant improvement in DFS.

Placebo-controlled clinical trials to explore this area were stopped when the comparative benefit of the aromatase inhibitor became clear. So the questions of how long to extend adjuvant treatment with an aromatase inhibitor after 5 years of tamoxifen or when the aromatase inhibitor should be started in relation to tamoxifen remain unanswered. In the trials, patients started an aromatase inhibitor any time after they had taken tamoxifen for 4 years. Some analyses have suggested that patients may still benefit even if there is an interval of up to 12 months after completion of tamoxifen; these analyses could, however, be completely explained by a simple selection bias and there may be no benefit.

Side effects. Aromatase inhibitors have a different side effect profile to tamoxifen (Table 6.3). Hot flashes and gynecologic problems

TABLE 6.3

Side effects of aromatase inhibitors versus tamoxifen

Side effect	ATAC trial (anastrozole vs tamoxifen)	BIG 1-98 (letrozole vs tamoxifen)
Vasomotor (hot flashes)	↓	↓
Fracture	↑ (on treatment) (2.93% vs 1.9%)	↑ (on treatment) (8.6% vs 5.3%)
Bone density	↓	↓
Arthralgia/myalgia	↑	↑
Gynecologic	↓	↓
Thrombosis/embolism	↓	↓
Coronary	Similar	Similar
Cardiovascular	↓	Similar

ATAC, Arimidex, Tamoxifen, Alone or in Combination; BIG 1-98, Breast International Group 1-98

(bleeding or discharge needing medical assessment) are less of a problem, but patients may experience arthralgia/myalgia and a fall in bone mineral density, which may contribute to osteoporosis and fracture risk. The fracture risk is present only *while* the patient is taking the aromatase inhibitor and is probably seen only in women who had reduced bone mineral density before treatment. There are data to indicate that aromatase inhibitors do not have adverse effects on bone mineral density in patients with a normal bone mineral density before treatment. Women in whom treatment with an aromatase inhibitor is planned should undergo a baseline bone mineral density assessment and, if it is abnormal, it should be repeated after 12–18 months and intervention with calcium and vitamin D, and bisphosphonates considered. Women with established osteoporosis before endocrine treatment may be best served by a planned sequence of tamoxifen followed by an aromatase inhibitor, as bone mineral density may actually stabilize or improve during tamoxifen treatment because of its osteopenic activity.

Selection. There is little doubt that postmenopausal women with ER-positive breast cancer should receive an aromatase inhibitor as part of their adjuvant therapy; this is emphasized by the American Society of Clinical Oncology (ASCO) guidelines published in 2005. It could be argued that an aromatase inhibitor should be an upfront treatment as some patients (particularly those at high risk) may relapse early and, if denied an aromatase inhibitor for 2–3 years, may not get the opportunity to benefit. Conversely, patients with ER-positive disease may be at low and protracted risk of relapse and may therefore benefit from more protracted therapy; at present, this would be tamoxifen followed by an aromatase inhibitor, as there are no data to support the use of aromatase inhibitor monotherapy for more than 5 years. Economics may also be a consideration, as aromatase inhibitors are currently much more expensive than tamoxifen, and patient preference and co-morbidity (e.g. osteoporosis) should be taken into account. The gynecologic side-effect profile of tamoxifen may also influence the decision in favor of aromatase inhibitors, as significantly fewer gynecologic interventions are required.

Ovarian suppression/ovarian ablation

Beatson's landmark series of surgical castration by oophorectomy in 1896 followed, half a century later, by the description of surgical adrenalectomy by Huggins et al. were both empirical observations of the ability of estrogen depletion to arrest breast cancer growth. Since then, concentrated effort by endocrinologists and clinicians to understand and exploit these mechanisms has been important. Interest in ovarian ablation has continued. This was initially based on the observation that, in the early adjuvant chemotherapy trials, the level of benefit was higher in premenopausal women compared with postmenopausal women. This raised the possibility that part of the benefit of chemotherapy in younger women might be related to ovarian suppression, as it was also noted that premenopausal women who developed amenorrhea following chemotherapy appeared to do better than women who did not develop amenorrhea. It was thought that this was part of the mechanism of the effect of chemotherapy.

Reversible ovarian suppression can be achieved medically using gonadotropin-releasing hormone (GnRH) analogs, which downregulate gonadotropin release from the pituitary gland through effects on the lutenizing hormone-releasing hormone receptor. The first GnRH analog was goserelin, which was found to produce equivalent effects to surgical castration or radiation-induced menopause, in terms of inducing remission, in women with metastatic breast cancer. The highly reversible effects of goserelin and similar drugs allow young women the opportunity to regain menses after completion of therapy.

A number of clinical trials have been designed to investigate the effectiveness of GnRH analogs in the adjuvant treatment of breast cancer. Some trials compared the effectiveness of drugs, such as goserelin, with chemotherapy and, in these studies, goserelin was found to be equivalent to chemotherapy using cyclophosphamide, methotrexate and 5-fluorouracil (CMF). However, CMF is not regarded as a modern standard chemotherapy regimen and, for most women, goserelin would not be regarded as a substitute. A further generation of trials compared combination therapy with tamoxifen plus goserelin with tamoxifen plus chemotherapy. These trials demonstrated that a combination of ovarian suppression and tamoxifen may be equivalent to a first-generation chemotherapy regimen with CMF alone.

With the advent of second- and third-generation chemotherapy regimens, using anthracyclines and taxanes, the role of ovarian suppression needs further investigation. The Zoladex In Premenopausal Patients (ZIPP) trial indicated that ovarian suppression may add to the benefit of chemotherapy and tamoxifen in younger premenopausal women (aged < 40 years), but not in older women. A GnRH analog may be recommended in women who decline chemotherapy and could be considered instead of tamoxifen in women who may wish to conceive later. The use of GnRH analogs in combination with aromatase inhibitors is also under investigation.

Chemotherapy

The development of adjuvant chemotherapy followed the recognition of the effectiveness of chemotherapy in metastatic cancer and started with CMF-based regimens in the 1970s. A pivotal randomized trial by Bonnadonna et al. confirmed the survival advantage in women given adjuvant CMF over women who did not receive it. This was true for both pre- and postmenopausal women and the benefit has been sustained over 20 years of follow-up. Subsequently, the benefit of chemotherapy has been confirmed in many randomized controlled trials. Furthermore, as drugs were shown to be effective in metastatic breast cancer, they were introduced into the treatment of early breast cancer. In this way, the anthracyclines and taxanes have become a part of the modern management of early breast cancer.

The benefit of adjuvant chemotherapy has been established in meta-analyses. In a review of 15-year survival data from more than 150 000 women in more than 200 randomized controlled trials, it was determined that anthracycline-based chemotherapy could reduce annual breast cancer mortality by 38% in women aged under 50 years and by 20% in women aged 50–69 years. For women with hormone-receptor-positive disease, the combination of endocrine treatment and chemotherapy could, therefore, reduce mortality by almost 50%.

Evolution of chemotherapy. Most initial research was conducted with chemotherapy based on alkylating agents (e.g. cyclophosphamide) and antimetabolites (e.g. methotrexate and 5-fluorouracil). The first study, reported in 1975, showed that 12 cycles of CMF improved 5-year DFS by 19%. Subsequent studies compared treatment for 6 months and 12 months, and both periods appeared to be equivalent. Following this, studies of chemotherapy of even shorter duration were carried out, but a comparison of CMF for 3 months and 6 months indicated that 6 months was probably better in terms of 5-year DFS for women under 40 years and for women with hormone-receptor-negative disease; however, this study did not show superiority of treatment for 6 months for the population as a whole. Treatment of longer duration (12 months) is poorly tolerated. Some studies have used perioperative chemotherapy with only one cycle of CMF, but this is not a standard approach. Currently available regimens employ either intravenous CMF or oral CMF. The intravenous regimen comprises:
- cyclophosphamide 600 mg/m^2 i.v. on days 1 and 8
- methotrexate 40 mg/m^2 i.v on days 1 and 8
- 5-fluorouracil 600 mg/m^2 i.v. on days 1 and 8.

In the oral regimen, intravenous cyclophosphamide on days 1 and 8 is replaced by 100–150 mg/day orally for 14 days. Six doses of folinic acid (also known as leucovorin) may be given starting 24 hours after chemotherapy to ameliorate methotrexate toxicity, such as mucositis and diarrhea. As this regimen contains cyclophosphamide, an alkylating agent, it is very likely to affect fertility.

The addition of other drugs, such as vinca alkaloids (e.g. vincristine), have been evaluated in combination with CMF, but showed no additional benefit. CMF can be used in sequential regimens following anthracyclines (see below). The CMF trials established that dose is important and a fall below 85% of the planned dose leads to a reduction in 10-year overall survival, with patients treated at the lowest dose levels having the worst outcome. These trials were, however, confounded by other variables; for example, patients receiving a lower dose may have had poorer performance status and thus an inherently worse outcome.

Anthracyclines (e.g. doxorubicin and epirubicin) are the mainstay of most modern adjuvant regimens. The 2000 EBCTCG analysis confirmed the benefit of anthracycline-based chemotherapy over non-anthracycline-based chemotherapy (e.g. CMF) in terms of both DFS and overall survival, and was reinforced by the updated meta-analysis in 2005–2006. A number of adjuvant regimens are in common use:
- doxorubicin and cyclophosphamide for 4–6 cycles every 21 days
- 5-fluorouracil, doxorubicin and cyclophosphamide for 6 cycles every 21 days
- 5-fluorouracil, epirubicin and cyclophosphamide for 6 cycles every 21 days.

The absolute difference in survival in favor of anthracyclines is approximately 3%. This has to be set against greater toxicity with a higher rate of alopecia, emesis, leukopenia and infection, mucositis and diarrhea with anthracycline regimens compared with CMF. Data are emerging to show that anthracyclines may be particularly important in patients who have over-expression of *HER2* and topoisomerase 2α genes, which are both found on chromosome 17.

The recognition that a reduction in the dose intensity of planned CMF regimens (< 85% planned dose) is associated with an inferior prognosis, together with mathematical modeling, which indicates that the benefit of chemotherapy might be increased by increasing dose intensity, led to a generation of trials looking at higher-dose chemotherapy and more dose-intense chemotherapy. Dose intensity can be increased by either increasing the dose of individual drugs and keeping the same schedule (usually 21 days), or by reducing the interval between treatment (to 14 days) by using hematopoietic growth factors to stimulate early white cell recovery.

There are no convincing data to support dose escalation above so-called standard doses, which for doxorubicin would be 60 mg/m^2 in a 3-weekly cycle and for epirubicin 100 mg/m^2. Many clinicians use epirubicin at lower doses (60 mg/m^2 or 75 mg/m^2); however, the only trials investigating dose have demonstrated that 100 mg/m^2 is superior to 50 mg/m^2, and no data on intermediate doses are available. Trials of very high dose chemotherapy with autologous bone marrow or stem cell rescue as adjuvant treatment were carried out in the 1990s. Despite initial enthusiasm, an overview analysis of 15 trials has not confirmed any benefit for this strategy, even in women at very high risk in terms of survival, though a modest benefit (HR 0.87; 95% CI 0.81–0.94) in DFS was observed.

Dose intensity can also be increased by reducing the dose interval to 2 weeks. A randomized trial comparing 2-weekly dose-dense chemotherapy with doxorubicin and cyclophosphamide followed by paclitaxel with the same drugs given in a 3-weekly regimen found that dose-dense treatment was superior in terms of both DFS and overall survival. The results did not, however, hold true for the patient population as a whole and, indeed, no obvious benefit was seen in patients with ER-positive disease.

Taxanes. Two taxanes are in common use: paclitaxel and docetaxel. An overview analysis of taxane trials has confirmed the benefit of these drugs over anthracycline treatment alone, but debate continues as to whether this benefit is equal for the population as a whole or whether some women benefit more than others. Most of the trials have involved women at relatively high risk (e.g. node-positive patients), though some have included high-risk node-negative patients. There is some concern that patients with ER-positive disease derive less benefit than patients with ER-negative disease. This may lead to different regimens being employed according to perceived risk level.

Targeted treatment

Trastuzumab (Herceptin). Following the success of trastuzumab in prolonging survival in women with HER2-positive metastatic breast cancer, it is now being evaluated in four large multicenter randomized trials of early breast cancer. Overall, 13 000 women have been enrolled and the interim results were reported in 2005. These trials showed a significant benefit of treatment with trastuzumab for 12 months at 2-year follow-up. The reduction in the risk of recurrence was over 50% and in the risk of death between 26% and 40% (Figure 6.4).

The incidence of cardiac toxicity was low with a cumulative incidence below 4% and no cardiac problems emerged after completion of trastuzumab therapy. Cardiac monitoring of left ventricular ejection fraction remains essential.

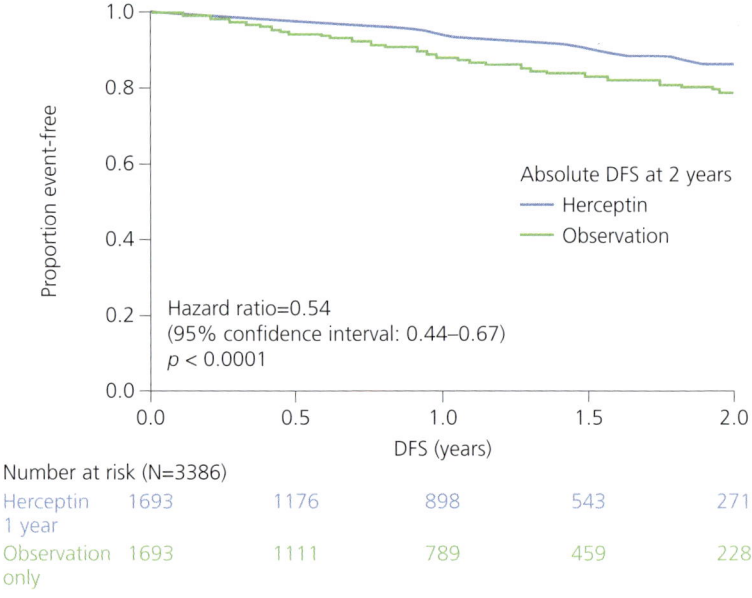

Figure 6.4 Effect of trastuzumab on disease-free survival (DFS).

Important questions remain, particularly relating to the duration of trastuzumab treatment. Indeed, a further trial (Finland Herceptin, FinHER) has explored adjuvant treatment with trastuzumab for only 9 weeks in combination with docetaxel and vinorelbine, and showed a progression-free survival of the same magnitude as that seen with trastuzumab for 12 months in the earlier larger trials. A number of trials investigating trastuzumab treatment for 6 months or less are ongoing, but the results will be important because this regimen would be less expensive and more convenient for patients.

Lapatinib (Tykerb/Tyverb) is a tyrosine inhibitor directed at downstream signaling for HER2. It is established for use in metastatic breast cancer (see Chapter 8), and is under investigation as a single agent and in combination with trastuzumab in adjuvant treatment.

Bevacizumab (Avastin) targets vascular endothelial growth factor, is established for use in metastatic breast cancer (see Chapter 8) and is undergoing trial as adjuvant treatment.

Bisphosphonates

A number of trials have evaluated bisphosphonates in addition to standard adjuvant therapy to establish whether they reduce the incidence of bone and other metastases. Initial trials with first-generation bisphosphonates (oral clodronate) were not conclusive. Recent trials of a newer bisphosphonate (zoledronate) have been encouraging in pre- and postmenopausal women with ER-positive breast cancer. The most recent results of an Austrian study have clearly shown a survival advantage from the addition of zoledronate to conventional systemic therapy. This is interesting, not only as it identifies another effective systemic therapy, but because biologically this is the first time that a drug that alters the internal milieu (rather than killing cancer cells) has been shown to improve outcome.

Making the choice of treatment

The decision to offer adjuvant therapy is complex and takes into account:

- the best treatment according to the literature
- treatment interactions with co-morbidity in an individual patient
- patient preference
- economic climate and national guidelines.

Some general rules of thumb, as starting points, are:
- hormone therapy reduces the proportionate risk of recurrence by approximately 40% in patients who are ER-positive or progesterone positive
- chemotherapy reduces the proportionate risk of recurrence by approximately 33% with CMF and up to 40–50% with newer chemotherapy regimens
- the addition of chemotherapy and hormones (sequentially) provides an additional benefit of approximately 15%
- patients with HER2-positive breast cancer should receive HER2-targeted therapy (currently trastuzumab) in addition to chemotherapy (± endocrine therapy)
- the risk for an additional patient is an absolute risk, not a relative risk (see Chapter 2); population estimates of proportionate benefit must be converted to estimates of absolute benefit for each individual, which can then be set against treatment for risk.

Adjuvant! Online (www.adjuvantonline.com) is a web-based program that estimates the absolute benefit of adjuvant systemic treatment for an individual woman; it may, however, be too optimistic for patients with adverse prognostic factors and younger patients (≤ 30 years). Adjuvant! Online is being updated to provide estimates of the benefit of trastuzumab for individual patients and Adjuvant! Genomic version 7.0 enables patients with node-negative/ER-positive breast cancer in whom a genomic score (Oncotype DX) is available to reach a decision.

Side effects. Cytotoxic drugs are associated with a number of side effects. Some are generic and common to most chemotherapy drugs (e.g. emesis, leukopenia, alopecia, mucositis, gastrointestinal upset and fatigue). Others are more specific to individual drugs. For example, taxanes are associated with sensorimotor neuropathy and myalgia, as well as skin and nail changes, which are uncommon with the anthracyclines. Anthracyclines can, however, be associated with cardiac

Key points – adjuvant therapy

- Adjuvant hormonal treatment and chemotherapy reduces the risk of recurrence of breast cancer by 33% and improves survival. The absolute benefit for an individual woman depends on her initial risk.
- For women with strongly estrogen-receptor-positive (ER-positive) breast cancer, endocrine treatment is the mainstay of treatment and the additional benefit of chemotherapy should be calculated.
- Women with human epidermal growth factor receptor 2 (HER2)-positive breast cancer should be offered anti-HER2-targeted therapy (provided there are no medical contraindications) as part of standard adjuvant treatment.
- Postmenopausal women with ER-positive breast cancer should be offered an aromatase inhibitor as part of standard adjuvant treatment.
- Taxane-based chemotherapy is recommended for women at high risk (node positive and high-risk node negative).
- Well-designed and managed clinical trials remain the preferred context for treatment.

toxicity leading to impaired left ventricular ejection fraction and, rarely, cardiomyopathy. There is a lifetime cumulative dose of anthracyclines, which should not be exceeded, and caution should be exercised in patients with cardiac risk factors, such as hypertension, obesity and diabetes. Hemotopoietic growth factors may be used as primary or secondary prophylaxis to minimize the risks of infection associated with leukopenia. The ASCO guidelines recommend that primary prophylaxis should be considered for all patients in whom a drug is expected to have an incidence of neutropenia of 20% or more and, in practice, this would include most patients receiving adjuvant taxanes.

Fertility may be a concern to younger women, especially as the average age of first pregnancy in the Western world is increasing. The risk of infertility with adjuvant treatment depends on ovarian reserve, which is related to the age of the woman. For example, permanent amenorrhea and infertility are rare in women aged 30 years and below, but high (> 80%) in women over 40 years. This may, in part, be related to the choice of regimen, with higher rates of infertility seen with more intensive regimens and in regimens employing alkylating agents, such as cyclophosphamide. Women should be given an opportunity to consult with a fertility specialist, if possible, before starting treatment to discuss the pros and cons of fertility preservation. Currently, the only proven method is in vitro fertilization with embryo cryopreservation. There is, however, considerable interest in the use of GnRH analogs to 'rest' the ovaries during chemotherapy and allow menses to resume thereafter. Unfortunately, few data on this approach are available and there are uncertainties about safety, particularly in relation to ER-positive breast cancers.

Key references

ATAC Trialists Group. Effect of anastrozole and tamoxifen as adjuvant treatment for early-stage breast cancer: 100-month analysis of the ATAC trial. *Lancet* 2008;9: 45–53.

Citron ML, Berry DA, Cirrincione C et al. Randomised trial of dose-dense vs conventionally scheduled and sequential vs concurrent combination chemotherapy as post-operative adjuvant treatment of node-positive primary breast cancer: First report of inter group trial C9741/cancer and leukaemia group B trial 9741. *J Clin Oncol* 2003;21:1431–9.

Coates AS, Keshaviah A, Thürlimann B et al. Five years of letrozole compared with tamoxifen as initial adjuvant therapy for postmenopausal women with endocrine-responsive early breast cancer: update of study BIG 1-98. *J Clin Oncol* 2007;25:486–92.

Coombes RC, Kilburn LS, Snowdon CS et al. Survival and safety of exemestane vs tamoxifen after 2–3 years' tamoxifen treatment (Intergroup Exemestane Study): a randomised controlled trial. *Lancet* 2007;369:559–70.

Early Breast Cancer Trialists' Collaborative Group. Tamoxifen for early breast cancer: an overview of the randomised trials. *Lancet* 1998;251:1451–67.

Early Breast Cancer Trialists' Collaborative Group. Ovarian ablation in early breast cancer: overview of randomised trials. *Lancet* 1996;348:1189–96.

Eastell R, Adams JE, Colman RE et al. Affect of anastrozole on bone mineral density: 5-year results from the anastrozole, tamoxifen, alone or in combination trial 18233230. *J Clin Oncol* 2008;26:1051–7.

Gnant M, Mlineritsh B, Schippinger W et al. Endocrine therapy plus zoledronic acid in pre-menopausal breast cancer. *N Engl J Med* 2009;360:679–91.

Goldhirsch A, Ingle JN, Gelber RD et al; Panel members. Thresholds for therapies: highlights of the St Gallen International Expert Consensus on the primary therapy of early breast cancer 2009. *Ann Oncol* 2009;20:1319–29.

Goss PE, Ingle JN, Martino F et al. Efficacy of letrozole extended adjuvant therapy according to oestrogen receptor and progesterone receptor status of the primary tumour: National Cancer Institute of Canada Clinical Trials Group MA.17. *J Clin Oncol* 2007;25:2006–11.

Jones S, Holmes FA, O'Shaugnessy J et al. Docetaxel with cyclophosphamide is associated with an overall survival benefit compared with doxorubicin and cyclophosphamide: 7-year-follow-up of US oncology research trial 9735. *J Clin Oncol* 2009;25:4765–71.

Mamounas EP, Bryant J, Lembursky B et al. Paclitaxel after doxorubicin plus cyclophosphamide as adjuvant chemotherapy for node-positive breast cancer: results from NSABPB-28. *J Clin Oncol* 2005;23:3686–96.

Romond EH, Perrys EH, Bryant J et al. Trastuzumab plus adjuvant chemotherapy for operable Her2-positive breast cancer. *N Engl J Med* 2005;353:1673–84.

Smith I, Proctor M, Gelber RD et al. 2-year-follow-up of trastuzumab after adjuvant chemotherapy in HER-2 positive breast cancer: a randomised controlled trial. *Lancet* 2007;369:29–36.

Suter TM, Proctor M, Van-Veldhuisen DJ et al. Trastuzumab-associated cardiac adverse event in the Herceptin adjuvant trial. *J Clin Oncol* 2007;25:3859–65.

Winer EP, Huddis C, Burstein HJ et al. American Society of Clinical Oncology Technology Assessment on the use of aromatase inhibitors as adjuvant therapy for post-menopausal women with hormone receptor-positive breast cancer: status report 2004. *J Clin Oncol* 2005;23:619–29.

7 Follow-up and rehabilitation

Follow-up

On the basis of several carefully controlled studies including randomized trials in Europe and North America, it is now appreciated that most local or distant metastases present between the routine follow-up intervals. The 'lead time' achieved by a search for asymptomatic distant disease is of little value, as it contributes nothing to the survival or quality of life of the patient. A less interventional approach involves clinical follow-up with a history and examination every 6 months for about 2 years, and annually thereafter. For this approach to work, however, it is vital that the patient should be well informed and present promptly should symptoms develop.

It should be remembered that regular and intensive follow-up does not improve the success rates for treatment of a recurrence. However, it may serve other purposes. The patient's perceived need for follow-up may mean that visiting her doctor regularly for reassurance (even if it is sometimes proven false) will improve her personal well-being. Physicians may also gain more job satisfaction by regularly seeing so many patients doing well rather than seeing only those patients who have had a recurrence. However, neither of these possible benefits has been tested in randomized trials. It would therefore be prudent to explain to the patient that regular follow-up, though offered, is not necessarily of proven value. In fact, the National Institute for Health and Clinical Excellence has recommended follow-up for breast cancer patients should stop after 3 years in England and Wales. Scottish doctors can, however, continue to enjoy the visits from their patients for as many years as they please.

From a different perspective, because our understanding of breast cancer is continually changing, it may be important to follow-up patients for a long time, not only to continue treatment (e.g. extended adjuvant hormone therapy), but to assess and treat the long-term side effects of therapy, such as osteoporosis and cognitive dysfunction, and the late side effects of radiotherapy.

Mammography. The role of mammography in follow-up is somewhat controversial. However, previous breast cancer is one of the highest risk factors for developing a breast cancer. If it is well organised to ensure that anxiety levels are not raised, a follow-up could offer a sense of reassurance to the woman, especially when the result is given immediately. Of course, as with any screening activity, such mammograms may pick up small cancers that may never have grown. Modern digital mammography has the advantage of better resolution and lower radiation and may reduce inaccurate results and unnecessary biopsies.

Clinicians and patients alike have to be reassured that the risk of local relapse within the retained breast is similar to the risk of a contralateral breast cancer, which is about 4% over 10 years. The relative risk of dying from a contralateral breast cancer depends on the recurrence risk associated with the original tumor. It may be extremely small when compared with the risk of death from the original disease. For this reason, a policy of annual or biennial mammography, for example, might be a reasonable compromise, but the routine use of tumor markers or imaging tests in the search for distant metastases cannot be endorsed. None of these tests has a high specificity, and the patient can therefore suffer repeated false alarms. Moreover, even if the results are truly positive for asymptomatic metastases, this merely provides the patient with 6 months' additional notice of impending death, during which time the reintroduction of systemic therapy is of unproven value.

Rehabilitation

Patients undergoing surgery for primary breast cancer require rehabilitation to address the physical and psychological consequences of surgery.

Physical rehabilitation

Physiotherapy. Although the incidence of severe arm and shoulder disorders after mastectomy has largely declined with the reduction in radical procedures, minor nerve damage may still occur, and thus physiotherapy should be started as soon as possible after surgery.

A range of exercises can be used to improve arm and shoulder mobility. The patient should be able to brush the back of her hair and fasten zips at the back of her clothing by the time she returns home, and exercises should be continued after discharge from hospital. Physiotherapy can also reduce the risk of lymphedema after full axillary clearance. Elastic bandaging may also be useful, and the affected arm should be elevated whenever possible, particularly at night, and protected from knocks.

Breast prostheses. The use of an appropriate prosthesis is an important aspect of physical rehabilitation after mastectomy, and can also strongly influence psychological rehabilitation. A light, temporary prosthesis can be used for the first few weeks until the wound has healed. A suitable permanent prosthesis can then be selected from the wide range available, according to the required size, shape and adherence to the chest wall. New developments in materials technology have overcome many of the disadvantages of traditional silicone prostheses (e.g. Duette, which uses two different types of silicone to produce more natural movement, and Harmony, which has a silky surface). Many hospitals have a nurse or physiotherapist trained in the use of breast prostheses.

Psychological rehabilitation. Breast cancer imposes considerable psychological stress and trauma. The initial diagnosis and preparation for surgery can produce a period of emotional turmoil in which rapid mood swings are accompanied by immense disruption to the woman's lifestyle. By contrast, the patient may be euphoric during the immediate postoperative period, possibly due to relief of uncertainty and anticipation of a return to normal life. This initial reaction is, however, transient, and many women experience a period of shock and denial, followed by anxiety, about 2–3 months after surgery. Most women eventually develop coping skills, enabling them to live a normal lifestyle. Approximately 20–30% of women, however, have persistent psychological or sexual problems 1–2 years after surgery, compared with 10% of age-matched women without breast cancer. This does not seem to be related to the type of operation; anxiety and depression appear to be as common in women undergoing conservative surgery as in women undergoing mastectomy.

It is possible that while women undergoing conservative surgery are less concerned about the mutilating effect of surgery and perceived loss of femininity, they are more worried than mastectomy patients about the possibility of recurrence. Patients may also experience anxiety or depression in association with follow-up visits to the clinic, because of the fear that the cancer might recur. If recurrent disease is detected, the patient must again come to terms with the risk of death and the need for further treatment; major depression may occur in up to 50% of women with recurrent disease.

Psychological support is available from a number of sources:
- nurse counselors
- volunteers
- self-help groups
- national organizations.

Specialist nurse counselors can offer advice and emotional support throughout the processes of diagnosis and treatment, and can identify patients with psychological problems requiring treatment. It is important, however, that both the patient and the nurse recognize when such support is no longer needed; maintaining contact on a purely routine basis can foster a sense of being unwell in the patient, making her feel that she is unable to cope on her own. Volunteer groups, composed of women who have had breast cancer themselves, self-help groups and national cancer charities can also offer valuable help and advice to breast cancer patients and their families (see Useful addresses at the back of this book).

Key points – follow-up and rehabilitation

- Conventional belief in the need for intensive follow-up after treatment for primary breast cancer is being challenged.
- Attention must be paid to both physical and psychological rehabilitation.
- Simple physical exercises, initiated early, accelerate and improve rehabilitation.
- Short- and long-term emotional and spiritual support should not be overlooked.

Key references

GIVIO Investigators. Impact of follow-up testing on survival and health-related quality of life in breast cancer patients. *JAMA* 1994;271: 1587–92.

Rosselli Del Turco M, Palli D, Cariddi A et al. for the National Research Council Project on Breast Cancer Follow-up. Intensive diagnostic follow-up after treatment of primary breast cancer. *JAMA* 1994;271:1593–7.

These studies are now over 15 years old and, arguably, patients treated with newer systemic therapies may benefit from the lead time gained by intensive follow-up and the sensitivity of newer imaging modalities. A randomized trial to test the benefits and harms of this would be appropriate now.

8 Management of advanced cancer

Although metastatic breast cancer may develop after primary treatment of breast cancer, 5% of patients have metastatic disease at the initial presentation. Approximately 50% of metastases develop within the first 5 years after diagnosis, but the risk of breast cancer is lifelong and, counterintuitively, tumors with a better prognosis, such as estrogen-receptor-positive (ER-positive) tumors, may relapse late (i.e. 10–15 years after diagnosis). Patients with a poorer prognosis at the time of primary diagnosis tend to relapse early and have an inherently higher risk of relapse.

Although metastases normally invade multiple organs, 5% may present as a solitary metastasis. Women with a solitary metastasis are an important group as, with local surgical treatment or radiotherapy in addition to systemic treatment, they may become long-term survivors. Bone is the most common site for metastatic disease, followed by lung, liver and soft tissue. Brain metastases are not uncommon and, as patients survive longer, are becoming an increasing clinical problem. Symptoms of advanced/metastatic breast cancer are listed in Table 8.1.

Following diagnosis, metastatic breast cancer requires staging, which includes:
- blood tests (full blood count and biochemistry including calcium)
- computed tomography (CT) of the chest and abdomen (± pelvis)
- isotope bone scan
- other tests as required (e.g. radiographs of bones to assess fracture risk, magnetic resonance imaging [MRI] for suspected spinal cord compression)
- measurement of tumor markers, carcinoembryonic antigen and cancer antigen 15-3 are sometimes used either to help establish the diagnosis or to monitor response to treatment; their use is not established in the follow-up of asymptomatic patients following primary cancer diagnosis because of low sensitivity and specificity
- positron emission tomography-CT (PET-CT) is used in diagnosis and staging as it provides both anatomic imaging and a measurement of

TABLE 8.1

Symptoms of advanced cancer

Locally advanced disease
- Peau d'orange and infiltration of the skin and, occasionally, ulceration (because of blockage by involved lymph nodes [not postsurgical])
- Lymphedema with swelling of the arm
- Pain or paralysis of the arm as a result of nerve involvement

Bone metastases
- Bone pain or pathological fractures
- Spinal cord compression caused by spinal metastases
- Weakness and lethargy, nausea and vomiting, constipation and general malaise due to hypercalcemia

Lung metastases
- Cough
- Breathlessness

Liver metastases
- Nausea
- Anorexia
- Weight loss
- Jaundice

Brain metastases
- Headaches and neurological symptoms due to increased intracranial pressure
- Headache, nausea and cerebellar symptoms associated with meningeal disease

disease activity; in some cases, it may be used to follow the progression of disease, but this is still experimental.

Conventionally, metastatic breast cancer is incurable. However, the prognosis for patients with metastases has improved and about 20% of patients will be alive 5 years from diagnosis. It is important to have a clear view of the aim of treatment. In clinical trials, this is measured in terms of response rates, time to progression and survival; outside trials and in clinical practice, however, the benefits of treatment are more commonly assessed by relief of symptoms and maintained quality of life. It is important to consider patients holistically in light of their co-morbidities, social environment and their own and their family's wishes.

Metastatic breast cancer is increasingly a chronic and recurrent disease characterized by remission and relapses, but it can lead to oncological emergencies requiring immediate treatment (Table 8.2). In an individual patient, the best predictor of outcome is previous response. For example, patients with a long disease-free interval after primary treatment and good performance status, small volume disease and so-called 'favorable' disease sites (bone, soft tissue) are likely to do better than patients who relapse very soon after initial adjuvant treatment or who have poor performance status as a consequence of high disease burden and possibly multiple disease sites with visceral involvement (i.e. liver, lung).

Systemic treatment can improve symptoms in 30–70% of patients and may delay disease progression. With newer combination regimens,

---

TABLE 8.2

Oncological emergencies

Suspicion alone of the following conditions warrants immediate specialist attention
- Neutropenic fever (due to chemotherapy)
- Spinal cord compression
- Uncontrolled pain
- Cerebral metastases
- Incipient fracture of femur or other bone
- Hypercalcemia
- Jaundice (obstructive picture)
- Bone marrow failure (usually presents as anemia and/or thrombocytopenia)

particularly those given in combination with targeted therapy, there may be an opportunity to improve overall survival. For patients whose initial disease was steroid hormone-receptor-positive, the preferred initial treatment for metastases is hormonal, provided that the characteristics of the disease are not aggressive (i.e. long disease-free interval, hormone-receptor-positive disease, bone-only disease). Chemotherapy is reserved for steroid hormone-receptor-negative disease and disease that fails to respond to hormonal treatment. Patients with human epidermal growth factor receptor 2 (HER2)-positive disease should receive anti-HER2 targeted therapy as their main treatment, usually in combination with chemotherapy.

Endocrine therapy

Premenopausal women. Endocrine therapy in premenopausal women usually involves ovarian ablation, which can be done laparoscopically with minimal morbidity, or by using a gonadotropin-releasing hormone (GnRH) analog, such as goserelin, which can be given monthly by subcutaneous depot injection. GnRH analogs block estrogen secretion by inhibiting the release of luteinizing hormone. Local side effects may include pain or swelling at the injection site and patients also experience menopausal symptoms. Some premenopausal women may be offered tamoxifen. However, as this is usually the treatment of choice in adjuvant therapy, most women will have been exposed to tamoxifen and thus ovarian suppression (possibly with an aromatase inhibitor) is preferred for metastatic disease.

Endocrine therapy in postmenopausal women. Aromatase inhibitors are the standard of care as first-line therapy. Three aromatase inhibitors are in current use:
- anastrozole (non-steroidal)
- letrozole (non-steroidal)
- exemestane (steroidal).

Evidence from clinical trials has led to the recommendation that an aromatase inhibitor is the standard of care for the first-line treatment of postmenopausal hormone-dependent advanced breast cancer.

Most patients will relapse at some point following first-line hormonal treatment (median time 15–18 months) and, provided they have demonstrated a response or clinical benefit to first-line treatment, second-line endocrine treatment can be considered. Options include:

- tamoxifen (however, few data are available to validate the use of tamoxifen after an aromatase inhibitor, though response has been noted anecdotally)
- a steroidal aromatase inhibitor (exemestane)
- fulvestrant, which is a steroidal anti-estrogen that binds to the ER, reducing the number of ER molecules in the cell thereby downregulating this receptor and suppressing the expression of estrogen-dependent genes; this compound is a pure anti-estrogen and has no estrogen agonist activity
- progestins (e.g. megestrol acetate or medroxyprogesterone acetate), which are given orally and may be associated with weight gain, fluid retention and diabetes.

There is no consensus as to the optimal second-line endocrine therapy for postmenopausal women. Non-steroidal aromatase inhibitors are often used as first-line treatment and thus steroidal aromatase inhibitors may be used as second-line therapy. However, the response rates to exemestane in phase II trials are only around 10%.

Tamoxifen as second-line therapy. As aromatase inhibitors have moved to first-line therapy, both in the adjuvant situation and in metastatic disease, understanding the role of tamoxifen as second-line therapy would be helpful, but few trials have investigated this. The data available have shown that it remains helpful.

Overexpression of HER2 in hormone-receptor-positive breast cancer. Retrospective analyses of endocrine therapy in steroid hormone-receptor-positive breast cancer, with concurrent overexpression of *HER2*, have indicated that metastatic breast cancer with overexpression of *HER2* is less responsive to endocrine treatment, especially tamoxifen. This may be explained by 'in vitro' data, which have indicated that the presence of HER2 downregulates estrogen-receptor production, thereby rendering cells less responsive to anti-estrogen therapy. In a phase III trial comparing anastrozole plus trastuzumab with anastrozole alone as first-line therapy, progression-free survival was poor (< 4 months) in both treatment arms, though an improvement in progression-free survival in favor of trastuzumab was seen in the combination arm. In a phase II trial of letrozole and trastuzumab, the overall response rate to the combination in patients who had previously received tamoxifen was 26% with median time to disease progression of 5.8 months; however, a large number of patients in this trial also experienced early progressive disease, indicating overlapping resistance. A recent study of the oral tyrosine kinase inhibitor lapatinib in combination with letrozole has demonstrated superior response rates and time to progression in favor of the combination. There are several ongoing trials combining hormonal treatment and other targeted therapy with the anti-HER2 agent, farnesyl transferase, and angiogenesis inhibitors. It should be recognized, however, that patients with hormone-receptor-positive disease who have overexpression of *HER2* do badly and should perhaps be considered for chemotherapy at an early stage in their metastatic disease.

Systemic chemotherapy

Many cytotoxic drugs have activity in breast cancer. The choice of drug(s) will depend on previous adjuvant treatment, performance status, organ function and patient preference (Figure 8.1). Taxanes are recommended for patients previously exposed to anthracyclines and capecitabine is often used for patients previously exposed to both anthracyclines and taxanes.

Meta-analysis has shown the superiority of combination regimens, especially taxane-based regimens, over single-agent regimens, albeit with increased toxicity. Combination regimens are more commonly used in the USA compared with Europe, especially for the first-line treatment of metastatic disease. Single agents are used worldwide as second- and third-line treatments, but response rates are lower with successive regimens which are of shorter duration than first-line treatment and, at this stage, palliation is of increasing importance.

Drugs can be given, usually as a 3-weekly cycle, until disease progression or unacceptable toxicity, which is common practice in the USA, or for a fixed number of courses (often six), which is common practice in Europe. Weekly low-dose schedules may be used for patients with poor performance status and/or organ dysfunction. All

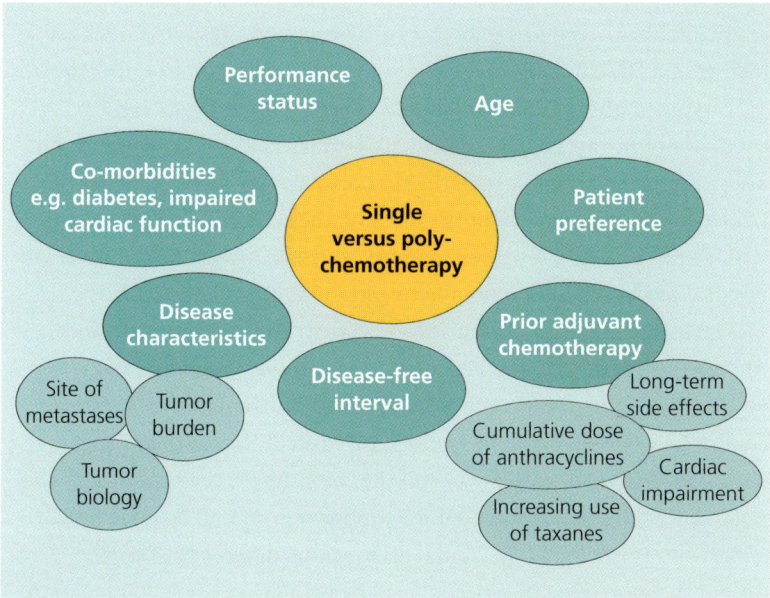

Figure 8.1 Factors influencing chemotherapy decisions in advanced breast cancer.

chemotherapy regimens should be given with modern anti-emetic cover using 5-hydroxytryptamine subtype 3 (5-HT3) receptor antagonists or substance P antagonists, with monitoring of both response and treatment-related toxicity. The use of primary prophylactic growth factors to maintain neutrophil counts is recommended for regimens with an expected neutropenic rate greater than 20%.

Targeted therapy

HER2-targeted therapy. Overproduction of HER2 can be identified by immunohistochemistry or fluorescence-in-situ-hybridization of the primary tumor. It is seen in 25% of breast cancers and is associated with an inferior prognosis.

Although nowadays many patients will have received trastuzumab as adjuvant treatment, those patients who relapse with metastatic disease should be rechallenged with trastuzumab as first-line therapy, usually in combination with chemotherapy (a taxane), either weekly or 3 weekly. While the chemotherapy is usually for a fixed number of courses, trastuzumab is continued until disease progression. Response rates are high with a 50–60% improvement in overall survival of around 7 months.

Trastuzumab has none of the side effects commonly seen with chemotherapy, but approximately 50% of patients will experience an infusion-related reaction with the first dose comprising fevers or chills, which can be managed symptomatically; these reactions rarely occur with the second or subsequent courses. Cardiac monitoring is necessary because of the potential fall in left ventricular ejection fraction.

The use of trastuzumab has led to control of systemic disease and the emergence of brain metastases. If brain disease progresses with no evidence of progression elsewhere, then trastuzumab should be continued while the brain metastases are treated. Recent data indicate that, if metastatic disease in visceral sites or bone progresses during treatment with trastuzumab, HER2 suppression should be maintained either with trastuzumab in combination with a different cytotoxic drug (e.g. vinorelbine or capecitabine), or with lapatinib in combination with capecitabine. Lapatinib is an oral tyrosine kinase inhibitor that blocks downstream signaling from the HER2. A number of other new treatments targeted against the HER2 have been developed, including pertuzumab.

Vascular endothelial growth factor. Bevacizumab is a monoclonal antibody against vascular endothelial growth factor-A, which inhibits tumor growth by blocking angiogenesis. It has been approved for use as first-line therapy in metastatic breast cancer in combination with weekly paclitaxel for patients with HER2-negative breast cancer. It should not be given in close temporal relation to surgery, because of the risk of bleeding, and patients must be monitored for hypertension, bleeding and proteinuria. The optimal duration of treatment (fixed course or until disease progression) is uncertain. Other drugs targeting tumor vasculature are undergoing clinical trials.

Other new agents. Identification of other targets in breast cancer has led to the development of many new targeted therapies, largely comprising monoclonal antibodies or oral small molecule tyrosine kinase inhibitors, which are currently being evaluated in clinical trials

TABLE 8.3
New therapeutic approaches in breast cancer

Inhibition target	Example	Phase of development
HER2 dimerization	Pertuzumab	III
Farnesyl transferase	Tipifarnib and lonafarnib	I and II
Mammalian target of rapamycin (mTOR)	Temsirolimus Everolimus	II and III
Insulin-like growth factor	AEW-S41 ANG479	I
Tubulin	Eribulin	III
Aurora kinases	CCT-1292002 AZD-1152	Preclinical/ phase I
SrC	Dasatinib	II/III
Multitargeted receptor kinases	Sunitinib Motesanib Sorafenib	II/III

either alone or in combination with endocrine treatment or chemotherapy (Table 8.3).

Triple-negative breast cancer

Triple-negative (TRN) breast cancers are those cancers that do not have steroid-hormone receptors or HER2. They comprise 15% of breast cancers, but are more common in younger patients and in African-Americans compared with white populations, and are also more common in Arabic countries; this may reflect underlying genetic differences. TRN breast cancers have a predilection to metastasize to the liver and brain. TRN breast cancer has some molecular homology with breast cancers associated with *BRCA1*, most of which are triple negative and have a so-called basal phenotype.

TRN breast cancers may be more sensitive to chemotherapy, especially platinum-based drugs and taxanes. Drugs targeting VEGF, such as bevacizumab, and drugs targeting the epidermal growth factor receptor, which is produced at a higher rate in TRN breast cancer, are also of interest. A further class of drugs, polyADP-ribose polymerase inhibitors, are of interest in both *BRCA1* and TRN breast cancers.

Management of disease at individual sites

Locally advanced breast cancer or inflammatory breast cancer should be staged to exclude metastatic disease and then managed with systemic treatment, the choice of which will depend on a number of patient and tumor factors, including receptor status. Surgery may be possible after systemic treatment. Locoregional radiotherapy is recommended for all patients. Even if patients have small volume metastatic disease, local treatment of the breast is important to prevent problems associated with uncontrolled local disease.

Inflammatory breast cancer accounts for 1–2% of all breast cancers. It is an aggressive form of the disease that is characterized by erythema, skin induration and edema, with or without a palpable mass. The tumor involves the dermal lymphatics, and lymph-node and distant metastases are common. Most cases have overproduction of HER2 and therefore require appropriate targeted therapy with trastuzumab and chemotherapy initially, followed by mastectomy and radiotherapy.

Bone metastases occur in over 70% of patients with metastatic breast cancer and may be solitary or multiple. They are usually identified because of pain or during staging after metastatic disease has been identified at other sites. An isotope bone scan with plain radiographs can be used to identify bone destruction and MRI to determine the cause of any neurological symptoms. Management is outlined in Table 8.4.

If a metastasis in the femur or humerus has destroyed more than 50% of the cortical bone or the patient is in severe pain, prophylactic internal fixation is advisable. This should be followed by radiotherapy. Similarly, patients with spinal cord compression should be considered for surgical decompression, if appropriate (e.g. one level only). Painful spinal lesions may be managed by vertebroplasty or kyphoplasty, which are minimally invasive procedures in which a cement mixture is injected to restore integrity of the vertebra involved. Radiotherapy is used after surgical fixation or to treat spinal cord compression that is not amenable to surgery and also for localized bony pain.

> **TABLE 8.4**
> **Treatment of bone metastases**
>
> Always consider bisphosphonates
>
> **Localized bone pain**
> - External-beam radiotherapy
> - Analgesics
> - Non-steroidal anti-inflammatory drugs
> - Vertebroplasty
>
> **Pathological fractures**
> - Internal fixation and radiotherapy
> - Bone gels
>
> **Widespread bone pain**
> - Bisphosphonates
> - Non-steroidal anti-inflammatory drugs
> - Systemic treatment (endocrine/chemotherapy)
> - Opiate analgesia
> - Radioactive strontium*
> - Sequential hemibody radiotherapy*
>
> *Rarely used

Patients with symptomatic bone metastases should be treated with bisphosphonates to suppress osteoclast activity and inhibit bone resorption. In clinical trials, bisphosphonates delay skeleton-related events, such as pain and fracture. Both intravenous and oral forms are available, and the drugs are classified as first, second and third generation according to the order of development. Care should be taken to ensure normal renal function, and to adjust both dose and infusion rate if abnormalities arise. Bisphosphonates are generally well tolerated, though a small proportion of patients may experience infusion-related reactions. Concerns have also recently been raised regarding osteonecrosis of the jaw requiring major dental work in patients receiving third-generation bisphosphonates.

Hypercalcemia is becoming more uncommon in breast cancer, probably because of more active management of bone disease at an early stage. Patients may present symptomatically and should be treated with intravenous fluids and diuretics, together with bisphosphonates. If hypercalcemia is refractory to bisphosphonates, then calcitonin may be considered. Corticosteroids have limited use.

Pleural and pericardial effusions. Breathlessness caused by pleural effusion can be relieved by chest drainage before appropriate systemic treatment is given. For most patients, however, a video-assisted thoracic surgical procedure is preferable, both to drain the fluid and to perform pleurodesis. Pericardial effusions can be drained under imaging control, but may require a pericardial window.

Lymphedema may occur any time after primary diagnosis. The incidence and prevalence of lymphedema is expected to fall with the adoption of minimally invasive axillary surgery with sentinel node biopsy. Patients should be advised about the risk factors for and signs of lymphedema, and encouraged to seek help should it arise, as proactive management will minimize morbidity. Management includes avoiding and treating arm infections, compression sleeves, massage and bandaging.

Liver metastases. In patients with jaundice, it is important to exclude extrahepatic biliary obstruction, which may be amenable to biliary duct stenting before systemic treatment. Corticosteroids may relieve liver capsular pain. Management is predominantly dependent on systemic treatment; however, there is interest in local treatment with radiofrequency or ultrasound ablation if only a few liver metastases are present. Resection may be considered for solitary metastases or disease confined to one lobe of the liver; however, only 10% of patients have disease confined to the liver.

Neurological complications. The apparent incidence of brain metastases is increasing, especially in patients with HER2-positive or TRN disease, and probably as a result of improved control of systemic disease. Patients may present with headache or neurological dysfunction, and intracranial disease can be identified by CT or MRI. Gadolinium enhancement may be necessary if persistent nausea or cerebellar symptoms arouse suspicion of meningeal disease. If metastases are associated with edema, treatment with corticosteroids will be necessary before and during radiotherapy. Solitary metastases should be considered for resection before radiotherapy. Intrathecal treatment with cytosine or methotrexate usually requires placement of an Omaya reservoir and can be used by designated personnel only.

Palliative care and terminal disease

In the final stages of breast cancer, the palliative aim of treatment becomes paramount. Because the natural history of breast cancer is very variable, this phase may last a few days or several months. The most distressing symptoms of terminal breast cancer include:
- pain
- insomnia
- nausea
- constipation
- dyspnea.

Pain is often widespread, and may have several causes. Each site and cause of pain should be identified to allow the most effective analgesic to be given. Strong opiates can be used when the pain does not respond to simple analgesics or weak opiates; fear of addiction is unnecessary and, with appropriate dose intervals, continuous pain relief can be provided. Laxatives should be given concomitantly to prevent constipation. Insomnia and anxiety can be relieved with benzodiazepines, such as temazepam or diazepam. Dyspnea is an under-reported symptom in terminal disease, for which appropriate interventions are available and appreciated.

The World Health Organization has introduced the concept of the pain ladder (Figure 8.2) in the management of cancer pain. This concept involves the use of a variety of agents, ranging from simple analgesics to opiates, depending on the site and severity of pain.

Spiritual and emotional support. At best, modern medical treatment can postpone death from advanced breast cancer to a limited extent,

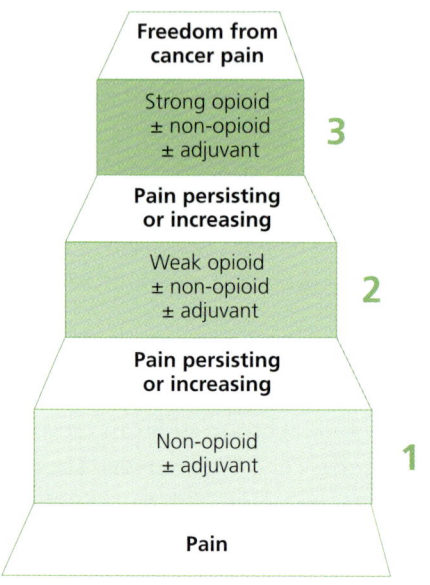

Figure 8.2 The pain ladder.

but there is a tendency to overmedicalize the terminal stages of the disease. In addition to symptomatic treatment, it is also important to remember the patient's emotional needs. Sooner or later we all have to recognize that, just as there is a time to be born, so there is a time to die. One of the greatest tragedies we can witness is the desperate patient, supported by her desperate relatives, seeking out magic cures at great expense in futile attempts to delay the inevitable.

It is essential that healthcare professionals recognize the need for spiritual and emotional support for the dying patient. While all doctors should, of course, be taught the skills of listening and counseling, no breast cancer team is complete without access to a professionally trained counselor or the appropriate ministers of religion. Coming to terms with the inevitability of death may have a calming influence and may even reduce the need for pharmacological support. The hospice movement, pioneered in the UK, is an example of this ethos at work and has now been copied in many countries around the world.

Key points – management of advanced cancer

- Site of recurrence, extent, time to recurrence and evaluation of co-morbidities are critical determinants of prognosis and treatment.
- It is essential to set explicit goals for both the patient and healthcare professionals.
- Systemic treatment can improve symptoms and, in some cases, prolong survival.
- Oncological emergencies must be anticipated and recognized.
- Effective pain management is almost always possible.

Key references

Alvarado M, Ewing CA, Elyassina D et al. Surgery for palliation and treatment of advanced breast cancer. *Surg Oncol* 2007;16:249–57.

Carrick S, Parker S, Wilcken N et al. Single agent versus combination chemotherapy in metastatic breast cancer. *Cochrane Database Syst Rev* 2005, issue 2. CD003372. www.thecochranelibrary.com

Coleman RE. Risks and benefits of bisphosphonates. *Br J Cancer* 2008; 98:1730–40.

Fallowfield L, Jenkins V. Communication of sad, bad and difficult news. *Lancet* 2004;363: 312–19.

Gligerov J, Lotz J. Optimal treatment strategies in postmenopausal women with hormone-receptor-positive and HER2 negative breast cancer. *Breast Cancer Res Treat* 2008;112:55–66.

Levy MH. Pharmacological treatment of cancer pain. *N Engl J Med* 1996;335:1124–32.

Nielson DL, Andersson M, Kamby C. HER2 targeted therapy in breast cancer; monoclonal antibodies and tyrosine kinase inhibitors. *Cancer Treat Rev* 2009;35:121–36.

Wilcken N, Dear R. Chemotherapy in metastatic breast cancer: a summary of all randomised trials reported 2000–2007. *Eur J Cancer* 2008;44:2218–25.

9 Clinical trials

The clinical trial process may be our most powerful analytical tool for developing and testing new treatments. There is also good evidence that the trial process itself raises the quality of care. However, a good trial must ask a good question and be structured to provide a reasonable chance of getting a good answer. Bad questions and poor execution defeat the purpose. It must also be remembered that no trial can supplant good clinical observation, the insight that develops a new hypothesis or the basic scientific discovery or technological advance that prompts the trial.

Should my patient enter a trial?

Many patients attending specialist centers are recruited into trials, and they often turn to their family physician for advice. Should they enter a trial? By all means, if the question is good, the design makes an answer feasible, and entry does not compromise the individual patient's care. However, clinical trials place a burden on all involved, because the data must be meticulously collected and analyzed; a good trial design will make this as easy as possible.

Trials can also be frustrating because the 'answer' will not be known until the study is complete. If your patient is one of the first to be entered into a trial with a 5-year follow-up, then – barring an unexpectedly dramatic result – you may not know the outcome for a decade.

Finally, an admission of uncertainty (a true equipoise between the two treatments being compared) by the physician is implicit in a randomized trial, which can be difficult for some patients (and physicians) to accept.

Characteristics of clinical trials

The purpose of a clinical trial is to conduct a human experiment that is likely to provide an answer to a clinical or a biological question (or both). Although there are regional differences in the extent of

informed consent required and its documentation, three fundamental principles apply.
- The trial must address a legitimate question to which the answer is currently unclear. In a randomized trial, this introduces the concept of 'equipoise', which means that each arm of the study has equal merit in advance of the experiment.
- The patient must be an informed and willing participant in the study.
- The patient may decline to enter the trial, or withdraw at any time during the study, without prejudicing their subsequent care.

There are four clinical trial structures, each of which has a different purpose.

The phase I study involves a small number of participants, and provides basic pharmacological and toxicological information. It is not a test of therapeutic efficacy. However, translational research can be performed in conjunction with phase I testing. For example, Bcl-2 downregulation by the Bcl-2 antisense oligodeoxynucleotide oblimersen in breast tumor biopsies was found in a recent phase I study. For drugs with relatively non-toxic mechanisms of action (e.g. endocrine agents), phase I studies may be carried out in healthy volunteers; trials on cancer chemotherapy agents are almost always conducted in major cancer centers and involve patients in whom all other available treatment has failed. Phase I studies are usually not randomized.

The phase II study uses phase I data to select a range of doses. The sample size is usually 15–20 patients, but may be increased if a major response is observed. The patients usually have end-stage disease, and may have previously received many other drugs. A phase II study may test drug combinations. Phase II studies are also performed to test newer approaches to treatment with (but not necessarily) new technology: for example, a phase II study of targeted intraoperative radiotherapy boost using Intrabeam found the approach to be safe, feasible, efficacious and with a lower than expected recurrence rate with long-term follow-up. Phase II studies are not usually randomized.

The phase III study is a randomized trial comparing the effects of different treatments, one of which represents the current 'state of the art'. Typical outcome measures are survival, disease-free survival, response, toxicity and quality of life. Because the differences in outcome between groups are often expected to be small, these trials involve many patients; they are conducted over several years and involve many institutions in many different countries.

The phase IV study is less commonly performed. Its aim is to evaluate the long-term consequences of an established treatment. In the pharmaceutical industry, such a trial might be referred to as a postmarketing study.

Manufacturers' trials may be performed to obtain regulatory approval, or advance the market position of the drug or device in question. Such trials are subject to the same ethical guidelines and constraints as other trials.

Clinical research groups' trials. The UK Department of Health has established a National Cancer Research Network (NCRN) to encourage clinical trial activity. One of its stated aims is to raise recruitment from 3% to 10% of eligible cancer patients; indirectly, this endorses the process as integral to good clinical practice. The NCRN can already boast a 7% accrual rate. This mirrors numerous national and regional efforts to accrue patients rapidly and advance clinical science. In the USA, there are several large clinical trials groups, including the Southwestern Oncology Group (SWOG), the National Surgical Adjuvant Breast and Bowel Program (NSABP), and the Eastern Co-operative Oncology Group (ECOG), to name a few. In Canada, the Canadian National Cancer Institute (NCI/C) is the leading agency. There are similar groups in Australia and in mainland Europe.

In recent years, even these large organizations have begun to pool efforts globally, both to increase the accrual rate and to advance the generalizability of the result. These clinical research groups are academically based, and closely linked to governmental research agencies. The compounds and strategies being tested come from laboratory research involving both public and private sectors. Generally the investigational agents are provided by the government or the pharmaceutical company without cost to the patient or institution.

Stopping rules

Patient safety is of primary concern in a trial. It is possible that a new treatment may harbor an unanticipated disadvantage or that treatments compared may have much greater differences in effect than anticipated. Such concerns are addressed by the interim analysis of blinded data, with rules to shut down a trial and make the results public if either of these events occur. These are not easy systems to design or execute. There is great pressure from all directions to get the data early. The risk is the loss of important long-term information. This issue is particularly important in the adjuvant setting, where much breast cancer research and treatment is concentrated. The controversy reached a public boiling point when a *Sunday New York Times* editorial called the early closing of an adjuvant aromatase inhibitor trial 'ethical overkill'. The trial designer must therefore give very careful thought to all the outcome considerations in a trial and to the early estimators that are used. It is our view that the referring physician, consultant and patient must understand these stopping rules, at least in outline.

Future of the trials process

The Human Genome Project and the study of derived proteins (proteomics) raise the prospect of ever more precisely engineered drugs. In the USA, a fast-track mechanism for cancer and other 'emergency' diseases has accelerated the introduction of new drugs. The trials process will thus gain even greater importance in the advance of medicine.

There will be consequences for every clinician's practice. For example, genetic prediction (e.g. *BRCA1/2*) will lead to proposed interventions before the disease even becomes apparent, and possibly before the early transforming event. Trials will involve large numbers of 'worried well', and will require long follow-up and expanded scrutiny for unintended adverse effects. Another consequence is that target groups will be smaller, so trials will become less centralized, raising questions about quality control and adequate surveillance.

Key points – clinical trials

- The well-conducted clinical trial remains the benchmark of both therapy and medical progress.
- The patient must be an informed and willing participant in the study.
- Patient safety is of primary concern in a trial.

Key references

Early Breast Cancer Trialists' Collaborative Group. Effects of adjuvant tamoxifen and of cytotoxic therapy on mortality in early breast cancer. An overview of 61 randomized trials among 28 896 women. *N Engl J Med* 1988;319: 1681–92.

Early Breast Cancer Trialists' Collaborative Group. Systemic treatment of early breast cancer by hormonal, cytotoxic or immune therapy. 133 randomised trials involving 31 000 recurrences and 24 000 deaths among 75 000 women (Part I). *Lancet* 1992;339:1–15.

Early Breast Cancer Trialists' Collaborative Group. Tamoxifen for early breast cancer: an overview of the randomised trials. *Lancet* 1998;351:1451–67.

Early Breast Cancer Trialists' Collaborative Group. Effects of chemotherapy and hormonal therapy for early breast cancer on recurrence and 15-year survival: an overview of the randomised trials. *Lancet* 2005;365:1687–1717.

Early Breast Cancer Trialists' Collaborative Group. Effects of radiotherapy and of differences in the extent of surgery for early breast cancer on local recurrence and 15-year survival: an overview of the randomised trials. *Lancet* 2005;366:2087–2106.

10 Future trends

A reconceptualization of cancer is now occurring: the idea of a relentlessly progressing, malignant *entity*, largely fixed in its properties, is being challenged by that of a complex, dynamic, ever-changing *equilibrium* of altered growth and metabolism. We suspect that the process we call cancer is a subtle, time-variable, non-linear regulatory process, and is probably field-dependent; in other words, a given molecule may upregulate in one setting, and downregulate in another. The implications of this conceptual change will be profound: if cancer is a potentially remediable disorder of regulation, its ultimate control cannot be achieved by killing all malignant cells, so the strategies used to devise new treatments, and the means of their evaluation, will also change. New drugs will achieve their effects not by killing cells, but by re-regulating them. Defective communication pathways will have to be reset or bypassed. Microenvironments that stimulate proliferation will have to be retuned.

We believe that most organs in the body produce latent cancers whose prevalence increases with age. These latent lesions, resulting from an accumulation of molecular events linked to a temporary failure of DNA repair, are a necessary but not sufficient condition for invasive cancer. They are sufficiently common in the breast, prostate and thyroid to suggest that all adults harbor cancer at some time. We think that, if left undetected, these cancers will exist in dynamic equilibrium with surrounding tissue for years until stochastic events, either adverse or favorable, lead to their progression to an invasive phenotype or return to normal. Adverse events might include further molecular damage, direct or indirect trauma leading to the activation of wound repair genes and angiogenesis, or even minor systemic disturbance such as may result from psychological trauma. Central to our understanding of this process is the recent work on pro- and anti-angiogenic cytokines, pro- and anti-proliferation cytokines, and pro- and anti-apoptotic signaling proteins. These provide a 'soup' within which a latent primary or metastatic focus can remain in a state of dynamic equilibrium, be triggered into progression or even regress to the norm (see Figure 3.2, page 33). There is a suggestion that it is perhaps the internal milieu of the individual that increases the risk of the development of malignant cells in several parts of the body, which supplants the conventional metastatic process.

Science is a search for understanding, rather than received wisdom. Professional acceptance of new ideas and changes in treatment cannot happen without dogged groundwork and consensus-building. Our understanding of breast cancer is a continuing odyssey. The description and categorization of fixed images and static parameters were an essential step, one that made the next step possible, in which we are coming to understand cancer as a dynamic process.

Prevention

On current evidence, we know that genetic predisposition plays a role in breast cancer. For some individuals, such as those harboring *BRCA1* or *BRCA2*, it is pervasive. For most, it is a small multiplier of relative risk.

Current preventive approaches reflect the anatomic consequences of the disease rather than genetic understanding (i.e. prophylactic mastectomy and oophorectomy). However, as the functional consequences of the genetics become clear, so will strategies to redress the mutation, such as drugs and advice on changing lifestyle to avoid enhancing behaviors.

Several population-based preventive strategies are emerging. Epidemiological evidence that delayed menarche, less body fat in adolescence and fewer ovulatory cycles over a lifetime lead to a reduced risk of female reproductive tract cancers has resulted in recommendations to increase youth fitness and exercise levels. As a considerably more interventionist step, work towards modification of the oral contraceptive is ongoing.

However, the tendency to intervene early in the cancer induction process will have to be tempered by the realization that, for every breast cancer that is prevented or delayed, many women will undertake treatment whose effects may not become apparent for a generation. Advanced disease may represent an end stage of the failure of control mechanisms in early disease, and thus be a very poor model for innovative therapy. In the short term, our zeal to identify risk factors must be tempered by the realization that therapies extrapolated from advanced disease settings may have only limited value.

One crucial question is how some women (a substantial proportion, in fact) are able to keep the microscopic cancers at bay for many years.

Early diagnosis

There is still much controversy over early diagnosis and screening. Even in postmenopausal women, the benefit is not as great as hoped (see pages 59–61). The anatomic approach to early diagnosis will eventually be superseded by tests that detect abnormal function. Genetic testing for susceptibility, positron emission tomography (PET) and PET combined with magnetic resonance imaging linking anatomy to function are early examples. Proteomics, the emerging study of the proteins produced by genes, may offer another approach.

Treatment

Several principles have been established in the treatment of evident disease, but their application has still to be optimized.

- Given good technique, less radical surgery with radiotherapy provides better cosmesis and a survival outcome equivalent to breast removal, though the local recurrence after mastectomy is slightly lower. Many women still opt for mastectomy; some because of the inconvenience imposed by radiotherapy. Newer approaches to radiation, such as targeted intraoperative radiotherapy, may relieve that concern.
- Broader use of sentinel node sampling provides adequate prognostic information without the consequences of full axillary dissection. As we shift from anatomic to functional staging, this requirement may also be relieved.
- Systemic treatment for breast cancer is now fully established. An expanded range of agents is available for hormone-sensitive breast cancers. Timing, duration and sequence will continue to be debated.
- For premenopausal women and cancers that are not hormone-sensitive, systemic cytotoxic agents remain the mainstay of treatment. The addition of the anthracyclines and taxanes to the established

cyclophosphamide, methotrexate and 5-fluorouracil regimen has increased the proportionate disease-free response rates by 10–15%. The trend is to extend the length of treatment, with enthusiasm for highly intensive therapies having been dampened by experience. Large trials will be required because the anticipated differences will be small.

The fields of molecular and genetic medicine are giving rise to a new range of options.

- Therapies aimed at altering the host side of the tumor–host symbiosis, for example anti-angiogenesis strategies, will become clinically available.
- Small molecules are being developed that are narrowly targeted to proliferation enzymes, such as matrix metalloproteinases, which have a role in invasion. Some 600 such compounds are in development.

Like trastuzumab, these drugs will be employed on a functional basis. Without doubt, the defining challenge will be when to treat and for how long. Do we intervene at the first expression of a precursor process or wait until a mass is present? It depends on the mode of action and efficacy of our treatment. The answers to the question require a fuller framing of the regulatory model. One scenario involves very early intervention for those at highest risk; tamoxifen and raloxifene are now included as an option for chemoprevention in patients at high risk of developing breast cancer. Later intervention would include the treatment strategy for small lesions that may be reversible (e.g. with anti-angiogenic agents).

Key references

Fidler IJ, Hart IR. Biological diversity in metastatic neoplasms: Origins and implications. *Science* 1982;217: 998–1003.

Fisher B. The evolution of paradigms for the management of breast cancer: a personal perspective. *Cancer Res* 1992;52:2371–83.

Index

abortion 12
Adjuvant! Online resource 102
adjuvant therapy
 radiotherapy 68, 71, 72, 73, 78–81
 systemic 22–3, 83–104
adverse effects *see* side effects
age
 epidemiology 7, 8, 9, 11, 28, 36
 screening programs 60
alcohol consumption 14, 15
analgesia 123, 124
anastrozole 91, 96, 115
anatomy 34–5
angiogenesis 33
blockers 101, 118, 119
anthracyclines 98–9, 102–3
anti-emetics 117
arm, postoperative problems 70, 72–3, 107–8
aromatase inhibitors 87, 96–5, 114–15
aspiration biopsy 57–8
ATAC trial 90–1, 92, 94
ATLAS trial 89
ATTOM trial 89
atypical hyperplasia 37
Avastin (bevacizumab) 101, 118, 119
axillary lymph nodes 35, 42–3, 52, 55
surgery 68, 69, 72–5, 133
Becker prosthesis 76
benign disease 35–7, 55, 57
benzodiazepines 123
bevacizumab (Avastin) 101, 118, 119
BIG 1-98 trial 91–2, 94
biopsy 54, 55, 58–9
sentinel node 68, 73–5, 133
bisphosphonates 101, 121, 122
black ethnicity 7, 119
bleeding
 from the nipple 48
 postoperative 70

bone metastases 29, 67, 112, 120–2
bone mineral density 94
brachytherapy 81
brain metastases 111, 112, 118, 122–3
BRCA1/BRCA2 genes 15–16, 119, 120
breast awareness 62–3
breast tissue
 density as a risk factor 12, 15
 malignant change in 30–3
maturation of 11, 12, 29–30
breast-feeding 12
calcitonin 122
Canadian Medical Association 62
capecitabine 116, 118
cardiac side effects 78, 100, 102–3, 118
chemotherapy
 adjuvant 22–3, 96–100, 102–4
in advanced disease 116–17, 119, 133
future trends 133–4
neoadjuvant 66–7
see also hormonal therapy; targeted therapy
classification
benign disease 35–7
cancer 37–9, 41–3
clinical examination 52
clinical presentation 38, 39, 47–9, 120
clinical trials 126–30
clodronate 101
clopidogrel 70
CMF chemotherapy 96, 97–8
COMICE trial 57
contraceptives 13

contralateral disease 57, 88, 91, 107
Cooper's ligaments 34, 38
corticosteroids 122, 123
counseling
 about risk 19–21
 treatment options 72, 75, 104
cyclophosphamide 97–8, 104
cysts 36, 37, 55, 57
cytology 57–9, 74
diagnosis 38, 39, 47–63,
112, 133
DIEP flaps 77–8
diet 12–13
dimpling of the skin 38, 52
docetaxel 99–100, 102
Doppler ultrasound 55
doxorubicin 98–9, 102–3
ductal carcinoma 38
ductal carcinoma in situ 30,
39, 40
ductal intraepithelial
neoplasia (DIN) 40
dysplasia 36, 37, 52
dyspnea 122, 123
ELIOT (Electron
Intraoperative Therapy) 81
emergencies 113
emotional support 108–9,
123–4
endocrine therapy 29, 66,
84–96, 102, 114–16, 134
endometrial cancer 89
epidemiology 7–17, 28, 36
epigenetics 17
epirubicin 98–9, 102–3
ESTEEM trial 66
estrogen receptor (ER) status
84, 86, 89–90, 95, 114
ethics 127, 129
ethnicity 7, 9, 119
etiology 30–3, 131–2
exemestane 92, 93, 115
exercise 14

138

International

The Canadian Breast Cancer Network
www.cbcn.ca

National Breast Cancer Centre (Australia)
www.nbcc.org.au

Wellspring (Canada)
www.wellspring.ca

Useful resources

UK

Adjuvant! Online
(Site designed for professionals and extensively updated in early 2004, aggregates data from many trials, particularly the Oxford Overviews, and provides patient-specific estimators of the impact of systemic interventions.)
www.adjuvantonline.com

Breast Cancer Care
http://www.breastcancercare.org.uk/

Cancerbackup
Macmillan Cancer Support
89 Albert Embankment
London SE1 7UQ, UK
Helpline (UK only): 0808 800 1234
Tel: +44 (0)20 7840 7840
www.cancerbackup.org.uk

Cancer Research UK
PO Box 123, Lincoln's Inn Fields
London WC2A 3PX
Tel: +44 (0)20 7242 0200
www.cancerresearchuk.org

Frenchay Breast Care Centre
Tel: +44 117 9753752
www.frenchaybreast.co.uk

healthtalkonline
www.healthtalkonline.org

Targeted Intraoperative radiotherapy
www.targit.org.uk

USA

CancerNet
NCI Public Inquiries Office
6116 Executive Boulevard
Room 3036A
Bethesda, MD 20892-8322, USA
Helpline: +1-800-4-CANCER
(+1-800-422-6237)
www.nci.nih.gov

The National Breast Cancer Coalition
1101 17th Street NW, Suite 1300
Washington DC 20036 USA
Tel: 008 622 2838
Tel: +1 202 296 7477
www.stopbreastcancer.org

Gnant M, Mlineritsch B, Schippinger W et al. Endocrine therapy plus zoledronic acid in premenopausal breast cancer. *N Engl J Med* 2009;360:679-91.

Liotta LA, Steeg PS, Stetler-Stevenson WG. Cancer metastasis and angiogenesis: an imbalance of positive and negative regulation. *Cell* 1991;64:327-36.

Schipper H, Baum M, Turley EA. A new biological framework for cancer research. *Lancet* 1996;348: 1149-51.

Schipper H, Goh CR, Wang TL. Rethinking cancer: should we control rather than kill? Part 1. *Can J Oncol* 1993;3:207-16.

Schipper H, Goh CR, Wang TL. Rethinking cancer: should we control rather than kill? Part 2. *Can J Oncol* 1993;3:220-24.

Sporn MB. Carcinogenesis and cancer: Different perspectives on the same disease. *Cancer Res* 1991;51:6215-18.

Vaidya JS. An alternative model of cancer cell growth and metastasis. *Int J Surg* 2007;5:73-5.

Fast Facts: Breast Cancer

phytoestrogens 13
pleural effusion 122
polyADP-ribose polymerase inhibitors 120
positron emission tomography-CT (PET-CT) 111–12
pregnancy, risk and 11–12
premenopausal women
epidemiology 7, 36, 40
treatment 84, 90, 95–6,
114, 133–4
presentation 38, 39, 47–9,
120
prevention *see* prophylaxis
progestins 115
prognosis 28–9, 38, 40,
43–5, 73, 112–13
prophylaxis 129, 132–3
prostheses 76, 108
proteomics 129, 133
pseudoangiomatous stromal hyperplasia 37
psychological support 108–9,
123–4
quadrantectomy 71
radiotherapy
brachytherapy 81
future trends 133
hypofractionated 79
intraoperative 69, 72, 79–81
in metastatic disease 120
postoperative 68, 71, 73,
78–9
raloxifene 87, 134
randomized clinical trials 128
reconstructive surgery 4, 69,
75–8
recurrence 28, 29, 33, 40
follow-up 55, 106–7
risk calculations 22–5,
65–6, 79
referral 49–50
rehabilitation 107–9
see also reconstructive surgery

research 126–30
risk, statistics of 7, 19–26,
61, 73, 102
risk factors 7–17, 28
Rosselli, Heath 4
screening 21–2, 29, 59–62
self-examination 62–3
sentinel node biopsy 68,
73–5, 133
shoulder, postoperative problems 70, 73, 107–8
side effects
bisphosphonates 121
chemotherapy 98, 102–4
hormonal therapy 89, 93–4
radiotherapy 78
risk calculations 23
surgery 70, 72–3
silicone gel implants 76
socioeconomic status 11, 52
spinal cord compression 120
staging 28, 40–3, 59, 111–12
START trials 79
stem cells 38, 67
stromal tumors 39
surgery 81
axillary 68, 69, 72–5, 133
complications 70, 72–3
conservative 68, 71–2, 80
contraindications 41, 67
future trends 133
mastectomy 4, 22, 57
67–70
ulcers 49
for metastatic disease 120,
122
oncogenesis and 33, 80
of primary cancer 66–75
reconstructive 4, 69, 75–8
tamoxifen
in primary disease 66,
84–90, 91–2, 94, 95
prophylactic 88, 134
as second-line therapy 114,
115
targeted intraoperative radiotherapy (TARGIT) 69,
72, 79–81

targeted therapy
as adjuvant treatment
100–1, 102
in advanced disease
115–16, 117–20, 120
future trends 134
taxanes 99–100, 102, 116,
119
terminal disease 123–4
terminology 40
thromboembolism 89
TNM classification 41–3
TRAM flaps 77
trastuzumab (Herceptin)
100–1, 102, 115–16,
117–18, 120
treatment
advanced disease 23, 67,
91, 112–23, 125
future trends 133–4
palliative care 123–4
planning 22–5, 41, 56–7,
65–6, 72, 75, 101–4
primary disease 22–3,
65–104
see also individual treatments
triple-negative (TRN) breast cancer 119–20
tumor markers 107, 111
Tykerb/Tyverb (lapatinib)
101, 116, 118
UK 7, 128
ulcers 49
ultrasonography 53–5
USA 7, 22, 128
vascular endothelial growth factor inhibitors 101, 118,
119
wide local excision 68, 71–2,
80
Xoft system 81
Zoladex (goserelin) 96,
114
zoledronate 101

Index

family history 10–11, 15, 22, 50
farnesyl transferase 116, 119
fertility 96, 103–4
fibroadenomas 36, 37, 39, 47
fine-needle aspiration cytology 57–8
5-fluorouracil 97–8
folate 12
folinic acid 98
follow-up procedures 55, 106–7
fractures 94
fulvestrant 115

gene expression patterns 45, 74
genetic testing 22, 129
genetics
cancer risk 7, 10–11, 15–17, 22, 119
tamoxifen efficacy 89
geographical risk 7–8
gonadotropin-releasing hormone (GnRH) analogs 95–6, 104, 114
goserelin 96, 114
hamartoma 37
HER2 see human epidermal growth factor receptor 2
Herceptin see trastuzumab
histopathology 38, 39, 57–9
history 51–2
hormonal risk factors 11–12, 13–14
hormonal therapy 29, 66, 84–96, 102, 114–16, 134
hormone replacement therapy (HRT) 13–14
hot flashes 89
human epidermal growth factor receptor 2 (HER2) 84, 89, 96, 115, 120
targeted therapy 100–1, 102, 115–16, 117–18
hypercalcaemia 122

imaging 52–7, 59, 111–12, 120, 123, 133

implants 69, 76
incidence 7
infertility 103–4
inflammatory disease
benign 36
cancer 67, 120
insomnia 123
intercostobrachial nerve 70, 73
intrathecal chemotherapy 123
Intrabeam system 79
Intergroup Exemestane Study 92
Japanese women 7

lapatinib 101, 116, 118
latissimus dorsi flaps 77
letrozole 91–2, 93, 114, 116
leucovorin 98
leukopenia 103, 117
liver metastases 112, 122
lobular carcinoma 38–9
lumpectomy 68, 71–2, 80
lumps 37, 38, 39, 47, 50
lung metastases 39, 112, 122
lymph nodes 35, 48–9, 52, 55
lymphoedema 48, 70, 108, 122

MA-17 trial 93
magnetic resonance imaging (MRI) 55–7
mammography 15, 39, 53, 60, 61, 107
Mammosite technique 81
mammotomes 58–9
management see treatment
mastalgia 47–8, 50
mastectomy 4, 67–70
menstruation 11, 28
metastatic disease 29, 39, 49, 83
staging 59, 111–12
treatment 23, 67, 91, 112–23, 125

methotrexate 97–8
methylation of DNA 17
Mobitron system 81
mortality rates 7
multidisciplinary teams 5
myocutaneous flap reconstruction 76–8

National Breast Cancer Coalition (NBCC) 60
National Cancer Research Network (NCRN) 128
NATO trial 88
natural history 28, 32–3, 39–40
neuropathy, postoperative 70, 72–3, 107–8
neutropenia 103, 117
nipple
discharge 48, 50, 52
inversion 38
reconstruction 78
nomenclature 40
Nottingham Prognostic Index (NPI) 43–5
nurse counselors 109, 124
obesity 12
oblimersen 127
oncogenesis 30–3, 131–2
opiates 123
oral contraceptives 13
osteoporosis 94
ovarian suppression 95–6, 114
paclitaxel 99–100, 102
pain
in advanced disease 120, 123, 124
symptomatic 47–8, 50
PAINLESS trial 66
palliative care 123–4
peau d'orange 48
pectoralis minor muscle 69, 73
pericardial effusion 122
pertuzumab 118
phyllodes tumors 39
physical exercise 14
physiotherapy 107–8

139